FIXING YOU™

BOOKS IN THE **FIXING YOU** SERIES:

Back Pain

Neck Pain & Headaches

Shoulder & Elbow Pain

Hip & Knee Pain

Foot & Ankle Pain

Back Pain During Pregnancy

FIXING YOU:™

NECK PAIN & HEADACHES

SELF-TREATMENT FOR HEALING
NECK PAIN AND HEADACHES DUE
TO BULGING DISKS, DEGENERATIVE
DISKS, AND OTHER DIAGNOSES

RICK OLDERMAN
MSPT, CPT

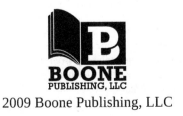

2009 Boone Publishing, LLC

Boone Publishing, LLC

Editor: Lauren Manoy (lauren.manoy@gmail.com)
Layout & Design: John Fellows (john@johnfellows.net)
Medical Illustrations: Martin Huber (mdhuber@gmail.com)
Exercise Photographs: MaryLynn Gillaspie Photography

Boone Publishing, LLC
www.BoonePublishing.com

Library of Congress Control Number: 2009900477

Library of Congress Subject Heading:
1. Neck Pain—Physical Therapy—Treatment—Handbooks, manuals, etc. 2. Neck Pain—Popular Works. 3. Neck—Care & Hygiene—Popular Works. 4. Neck Pain—Exercise Therapy. 5. Self-care, Health—Handbooks, manuals, etc. 6. Neck Pain—Alternative Treatment. 7. Neck Pain—Exercise Therapy. 8. Neck Pain—Prevention. I. Title: Fixing you: neck pain and headaches. II. Olderman, Rick. III. Title.

ISBN 978-0-9821937-1-6

Printed in the United States of America

Version 1.0

ACKNOWLEDGEMENTS

In science and medicine, we build on the shoulders of those who have discovered truths before us. Writing the Fixing You series has been no different. I would like to deeply thank Dr. Shirley A. Sahrmann for her breakthrough text, *Diagnosis and Treatment of Movement Impairment Syndromes*, on which the subject of this series is based. Were it not for her textbook and seminars, which I have immensely enjoyed, I would not have been able to write the Fixing You series, much less help so many people with chronic pain or injuries. Dr. Sahrmann is a rare breed of lecturer, therapist, and researcher with a sharp mind and wit to match. Her depth of knowledge in all things musculoskeletal and biomechanical leaves me speechless.

Additionally, I would like to thank Florence Kendall, Elizabeth McCreary, and Patricia Provance for their classic text, *Muscles Testing and Function*, fourth edition. This book has been a tectonic plate on which our understanding of orthopedic physical therapy stands.

THANK YOU!

I would like to thank Lauren Manoy for painstakingly editing this book. She has meticulously sifted through this information and helped me strike a balance between delivering technical information and making it digestible for you, my reader.

Thank you to Michelle for being my rehabilitation model as well as a star client!

Thank you Ken Margel and Scott Sturgis for shooting the rehabilitation video for me.

Thank you MaryLynn for the wonderful photos.

Thank you to Martin Huber for the illuminating medical illustrations.

Thank you to John Fellows for a fantastic design and layout.

Thank you to all my patients and clients who unwittingly served as my guinea pigs and those who wittingly modeled for pictures!

Lastly, thank you to my family for putting up with long hours of writing, meetings, and physical therapy speak.

This is dedicated to my wife Cecilia, my son Boone, and my daughter Edie.

CONTENTS

INTRODUCTION

*Thirty spokes converge upon a single hub,
it is on the hole in the center that the use
of the cart hinges.*

*We make a vessel from a lump of clay,
it is the empty space within that vessel
that makes it useful.*

*We make doors and windows for a room,
but it is these empty spaces that make
the room livable.*

*Thus, while the tangible has advantages,
it is the intangible that makes it useful.*

—LAO TZU

Fixing injuries requires, among other things, an understanding of anatomy and biomechanics. That is why this book and the others in my Fixing You series presents the Fixing You approach using clear and easy-to-follow language, case studies from my practice, and pictures and diagrams to guide you, the reader, in fixing your pain. My goal is to help you visualize exactly how your body works and what is going wrong when you experience pain. When you understand and can see clearly what causes your pain, you can develop and implement a plan to fix it using the exercises and tips outlined in the Fixing You series. But knowledge is only half the answer to the problem of chronic pain. True healing also requires adjusting your mental processes to work for you, not against you.

Attention to your body and how it is or isn't working is absolutely necessary to recover from chronic pain. In fact, lack of attention is a common factor in most peoples' health issues. Developing body awareness is often the most difficult—and most important—aspect of healing from chronic pain.

Intention is another intangible but crucial aspect of healing. Harnessing your intention—your singular focus toward getting better—will reap enormous dividends. Visualize it, verbalize it, write it down, and live as if you are getting better every day; in the process you will discover which habits are counter to your goals. Once you identify these habits, you can change them. Each change will reinforce your intention. The Fixing You series presents you with knowledge about the anatomy and biomechanics of injuries, and your attention and intention makes that information useful.

A NEW PERSPECTIVE

Since graduating from physical therapy school in 1996, I've spent hundreds of hours in continuing education classes and read countless professional journal articles and books that all attempted to answer these questions: Why do we have pain, and how do we fix it? I quickly realized there was more to injuries and healing than what I was taught in the courses I had been taking, although each had a piece of the puzzle. I realized that I needed a more complete understanding not only of how muscles and bones worked, but how they worked together to create movement.

Throughout my early years as a physical therapist, I tried one person's approach here and another's technique there. These various ideas about how to treat pain sometimes worked temporarily, but my clients didn't usually present or respond exactly like the case studies in the courses. Wanting to help people and not having the answers was frustrating. So I resolved to observe my patients closely, and I started to see the following patterns emerge:

- Patients resolving back pain using methods counter to traditional approaches.
- Chronic hamstring tightness and strains in athletes with strong hamstrings.
- Correcting structural issues in people with chronic neck pain and headaches only to have them return again and again.
- Knee pain in people whose leg muscles were strong and had good range of motion.
- Repeated straining of shoulder muscles in athletes whose musculature was strong.

In the meantime, I began exploring personal training over several years while working at an exclusive fitness club in Denver, Colorado. I had exercised all my life and found my work as a physical therapist limiting in terms of my career and life goals. Personal training seemed to be a natural extension of my interests in working with people within a larger spectrum than just treating them in a clinic.

My first client was a woman who was unable to raise her arm over her head. I reviewed her workout and found that she was doing all the wrong exercises for someone with her issues.

"Doesn't this workout hurt you?" I asked her.

"Of course it does," she replied. "Isn't it supposed to be painful?"

"No, it should be pain free," I said.

"What about 'no pain, no gain'?" she asked.

"No pain, no gain" is much like Nike's slogan, "Just Do It." You must understand that you still have to check yourself to be sure what you are doing is not harmful.

What may help one client may hurt another. I knew then that the fitness field needed more physical therapists. We are trained to not only assess joint and muscle function but to extrapolate that information into a performance model for sports, work, or just plain healthy living. Currently, the fitness industry includes personal trainers and Pilates, aerobic, and Yoga instructors who are trying to help clients in pain but who have limited knowledge of anatomy or the optimal biomechanics of a healthy body—much less an injured one.

Working as a personal trainer gave me access to a type of injury that I hadn't much experience with: chronic pain. As a physical therapist in a sports and orthopedic clinic, the majority of my patients had acute injuries or surgical repairs. But there are thousands of people—if not millions—in the clubs and corporations across the United States who are exercising or working in pain, fighting chronic injuries that they've been dealing with for years, and trying to make themselves better. I know because I quickly became the busiest and highest-producing trainer/therapist at the club during my tenure there. At the time, and even now to a large extent, most people do not have access to physical therapists' musculoskeletal expertise. I was seen as something of a novelty. Thus began my quest to synthesize a more complete understanding of how dysfunction and injuries were related.

A BREAKTHROUGH

As you are about to read, while treating one of these people, Debbie, I had an epiphany. Debbie had a 15-year history of neck pain and migraines after two back-to-back motor vehicle accidents, and she had tried everything and everyone to find relief. After a few sessions, I realized that her problem did not lie in her neck, but in her shoulder. I had made a critical connection that I previously hadn't thought about before: The structural damage the accidents had created wasn't the cause of her pain; it was caused

by dysfunctional biomechanics that created vu
which the accidents had exacerbated. We addres.
tional issues, and within a few days her pain had dis

Just as I was finishing with Debbie, I discovereα
confirmed my diagnosis and treatment approach with .
as a few of my other chronic pain patients. Written by D .ırley
A. Sahrmann, a physical therapist out of Washington University in St. Louis, *Diagnosis and Treatment of Movement Impairment Syndromes* is a medical textbook that provided the missing
link I had been seeking to pull together my observations. Many of
the biomechanical paradigms and rehabilitative exercises in the
Fixing You series have been adapted from Dr. Sahrmann's bril-
liant textbook. I recommend that all physical therapists purchase
the book and attend her courses.

Another book I regularly reference is Florence Kendall, Elizabeth McCreary, and Patricia Provance's classic, *Muscles Testing
and Function*. This textbook is a wealth of information for understanding precise musculoskeletal anatomy and testing. It is a stan-
dard in physical therapy, and I regularly refer to it for isolating
muscle testing. It guides me in specifically analyzing and thinking
creatively about function. By understanding muscle function on a
basic level, I can better hypothesize functional deficits that may
be occurring at a systemic level.

But my books are written for laypeople, not medical pro-
fessionals, to guide you in healing yourself. I've simplified and
distilled my medical training to reflect the majority of problems I've found when treating clients. I've prioritized the corrective exercises I've found most powerful for most conditions.
I've bolded vocabulary words and added information boxes to
help clarify words or concepts. I've also created videos of all
the exercises and tests to enhance the effectiveness of your program. To access these free video clips, visit my website at
www.FixingYou.net. Type in the code at the end of this book to
access the extra material.

HOLISTIC FUNCTION

The body is the sum of individual units working together to create functional movement. Bones, muscles, tendons, nerves, and ligaments can all be addressed individually, but it is important to understand how these structures work collectively to fulfill a purpose: pain-free movement of the body. So, while it is imperative that individual "chinks in the armor" are found and corrected, visualizing how the whole works together is just as important. This concept also works from the other direction; training movement and/or function reinforces and assists in correcting individual muscles' poor performance. In this book, I've introduced the key individual players—the parts that make up the whole—and also shown how they play together to create function, much like a symphony. You are responsible for bringing them in line to create your concert.

I wish you the best in your pursuit for solutions to your pain. You are not alone in your search for answers. I truly believe that, with a little thought and effort on your part, the Fixing You approach will help you find your answers, as it has for my clients.

The beauty of the body is that results happen quickly when you are doing the right thing. Most of the clients you will read about, and those that aren't included in this book, feel significantly better after only one or two treatments. Often, my clients understand they are on the right path within minutes of performing an exercise. Emboldened by this sense, they become more committed to the process of fixing themselves. You can have the same feeling of empowerment. There is no magical technique or device that will fix you. Only you can fix you—so let's get started on giving you the tools to do just that.

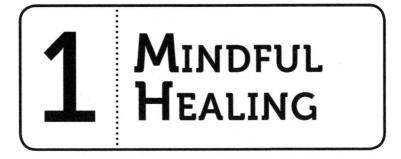

1 MINDFUL HEALING

There is not a single problem in LIFE
you cannot RESOLVE, *provided you*
first solve it in your INNER WORLD,
its place of origin.

—PARAMAHANSA YOGANANDA

Time and time again I see clients who have tried so many unsuccessful cures that they just don't know what to do. This is worrisome—not because I believe I can't help them, but because they don't believe they can help themselves.

The most powerful aspect of the Fixing You approach is that it shows you what is wrong, actually getting you to feel that certain muscles or movements are not working and how your pain changes when they are corrected. This helps define the problem. It gives issues a beginning and an end, allowing you to compartmentalize pain and therefore see when and how the solution will happen.

Given the tools to understand and correct your injuries, I hope you will feel a sense of empowerment that will motivate you to work harder to fix yourself. If you can define an injury, then you have the power to fix it—and that motivation will get you results.

Getting your head into your plan is essential. Without your commitment, chances are it will never get done. The exercises and techniques I describe in this book will only help you if you commit to them—or more importantly, if you commit to yourself. You cannot pursue any program halfheartedly and expect to get the big payoff. If I find myself more committed than my client, our work is done. I cannot want it more than them. In my experience, there are three processes involved with positive change: You have to visualize the problem and the change needed to solve it, verbalize your intention and write down a plan of action to fix it, and take action to implement your plan.

> Creating **positive change** involves internalizing your desire, verbalizing your intention, and acting on it.

VISUALIZE THE PROBLEM

Visualization of ideal movement is difficult for many people with chronic pain conditions. This is largely because they are unfamiliar with the anatomy of their injuries or the reasons their injuries exist. The information in this book will help you "see" what is at the bottom of your pain and how to fix it by giving you a glimpse into the underlying anatomy.

You will notice that as much as I discuss the anatomy of a problem, I also talk about movement. There is little use in learning anatomy if you don't also learn how it creates movement. You will learn what happens to your joints if your muscles are not working correctly and how that causes pain.

This brings me to another reason why visualization can be challenging. Most chronic pain is the result of years of poor movement habits—habits that have taken on the guise of "natural" movement, even though these are actually unnatural and harmful habits (also called **movement dysfunctions** or movement faults). For instance, you will discover that many people who experience neck pain and headaches have a poorly functioning shoulder blade. When the shoulder blade's function is restored, most people think, "That can't be right," followed almost immediately by, "Wow, my neck feels so much better like this!"

This tells me that their sense of biomechanically correct movement is actually wrong. What they "visualize" as ideal movement needs to change. To this end, I often ask my clients to perform their exercises in front of a mirror to give feedback on their form. Most people have never taken the time to observe their movement patterns, and this is a real eye-opener for them.

You may find that visualizing your shoulder blades' function will be more difficult than, say, visualizing your knee joint. Most of us have never seen our shoulder blades. To help you with this, look at a friend's or spouse's shoulder blade. Put your hand on it when the arm is down. Feel its borders. Compare what you are feeling to the pictures in this book. Ask the person to raise his or her arm while you keep your hand on the shoulder blade. You will begin to understand how it moves and how that movement corresponds to the images of shoulder blade landmarks in this book.

Then try it out on yourself. Have your friend feel your shoulder blades. Move your arms and get a sense of how they are moving. Feel their hands on your shoulder blades, and match this feeling with the pictures of ideal shoulder blade landmarks in this book. Once you get into it, getting to know your body this way can be an amazing experience.

You can practice visualization by closing your eyes and moving your arm or head in a certain way. With your eyes closed, picture where you think you've moved it. Then open your eyes. Is it exactly as you pictured it? Is the hand rotated the same way? Is your shoulder sitting as high or low as you expected? Is your head tilted a little more than you thought? Is your gaze looking higher than you imagined? Keep practicing this until your visualization matches your actual position. Have fun with it! You're exploring!

In the case of muscles that aren't working correctly, visualize them scrunching up and getting shorter when trying to contract them, and visualize them lengthening when stretching. Tap the muscle briskly to get it to "wake up." As you will see by my clients' stories, healing a muscle that has been under chronic stress can occur almost instantly. The muscles only need to relearn how they should perform. Pain will, in many cases, instantly diminish or be eliminated altogether.

> Set aside 10 seconds throughout the day to **get in touch** with your body and visualize its muscles.

Look at the illustrations of key muscles, and take some time to visualize where they are on your body and what they do. Using your fingers, feel the area in question to help yourself consciously connect with it. With your fingers on your upper **trapezius** muscle, for example, shrug your shoulder up or raise your arm overhead to feel this muscle contract. Connect what your fingers are feeling to what your brain is experiencing. Then try it without touching the muscle to see if you still get the connection.

VERBALIZE YOUR INTENTION

Solidify your ideas and support your intention to heal by talking to friends or family or writing down your plan. Often, discussing plans brings their fruition one step closer.

I think all of us have had a time in our lives where we secretly challenged ourselves to reach a goal but didn't tell anyone about it because saying it would heap more responsibility on our shoulders to make it come true. I've run into this situation countless times, where a client won't dare say they expect to become pain free for fear of not meeting their goal and being disappoint-ed. Even when they become pain free, they still doubt that it will continue. Take the plunge and express your goal or desire to elim-inate your pain. Put that responsibility on yourself. Hold yourself accountable for following through with this process of fixing your pain. Come up with a short phrase that affirms your intention, and repeat it throughout the day. "Every day, my body is working better and better" is an empowering statement that will help you keep a positive mental attitude. You can make this statement be-cause it is completely realistic, as opposed to setting an unrealis-tic goal, like running a three-minute mile.

Your body is not designed to be in chronic pain. Something you are doing or not doing is perpetuating your condition. Commit to yourself by telling your friends and family about your goals. By telling friends and family that you believe you will become pain free, you have already made a shift in your consciousness to believe that it will happen. Say it! Your friends and family will probably offer to help you in any way possible. This would be a good time to ask them if you can look at their shoulder blades!

So often in my life, when I'm working toward achieving a goal and getting hung up, I write about what I am doing and the problem I am facing. Write down your thoughts and experienc-es in a journal. Track your progress. If you're getting stuck on a particular concept or exercise, write about it. What is it that you don't understand? Where are you getting stuck? The act of writ-ing will help you see clearly where you are going wrong. It will also help you see what you are doing right and how far you've come since beginning to take action.

Write down how many hours (or minutes) of a particularly painful activity you can do before pain sets in. Write down how many repetitions of an exercise could be completed before you became fatigued. Check your progress in a couple weeks. Can you perform the activity longer before you feel pain? Can you do more repetitions before you experience fatigue? Have you learned a technique that eliminates your pain? Have you uncovered a habit that contributes to your pain?

All of these are great places to begin when tracking your progress. If you did something new that really hurt, then write it down. Figure out why it hurt. Make the necessary adjustments and see if those helped. On the other hand, if you found something that really helped, then write this down as well. It will be valuable information for you to implement later if you hit a plateau.

Create and write down two short-term goals like the following examples: "I will perform my exercises using correct form five times a day for the next week;" "I will set up 10 reminders at work, at home, and in the car to help me change my habits during the next week;" "In the next four days, I will identify 10 circumstances during which I notice a forward-head position."

Physical therapists use **short- and long-term goals** to create our treatment plans—and you should do the same.

Long-term goals should build on your short-term goals, like the following examples: "I will increase my exercise repetitions, using correct form, by 10 repetitions over the next four weeks," or "I will increase my exercise routine to include two strengthening exercises within three weeks."

TAKE ACTION TO IMPLEMENT YOUR PLAN

Finally, you must take action to reach your goals. I guarantee that if you do not take action, your goals will not materialize. So often, I give clients exercises to practice that clearly are instrumental in fixing their pain. When I see them next, however, I frequently find they've only performed one or two sessions since our last visit. This is not the most effective way to address chronic pain.

When you have a chronic pain condition, one repetition of an exercise each day will not fix it. Initially, you may have to exercise several sessions each day until the length or strength of the involved muscles are at least partially corrected. Once this is accomplished, your pain will diminish, and you can begin whittling down the exercises.

Often, a maintenance plan is necessary because movement

dysfunctions are what most likely got you into trouble in the first place. These will be more difficult to identify and correct because they are *habits,* and habits aren't easily broken. Throughout this book, I've offered some guidance for identifying common movement dysfunctions to help you recognize these and to get you started on correcting them. Ultimately, to permanently eliminate pain, these habits must be corrected.

Bringing your attention to what you are doing will be the most difficult aspect for many of you. In this book, you will find techniques and exercises to ease or eliminate your pain for good. You must, however, feel and notice how your body is moving and performing the exercises. Attending to your specific mechanics will deliver results. I see it all the time, and your body is built no differently than all the other people this approach has worked for.

With the demands of our busy days, it can be difficult to stay focused on these changes. That is why I recommend you set up a way to remind yourself of your new goals and to check in on your habits. Wear a special bracelet, ring, string, or rubber band around your wrist to remind you of the changes you are evoking in your mind and body. Place stickers on the dashboard of your car, the clock, your watch, your telephone—anything you use or look at frequently—to remind yourself that you are getting better every day by correcting those habits that feed your pain.

People often believe that they will have to permanently set aside a lot of time for exercise. Not true. I am asking you to make time over the next two to four weeks to heal yourself. If that doesn't sound realistic to you, then you need to rethink your priority of fixing yourself. Each session should take no longer than five to seven minutes, two to five times each day. In total, I am asking you to take 35 minutes a day for the next two to four weeks to get rid of years worth of pain. That doesn't sound too bad, does it?

THE MIND–BODY CONNECTION

A woman I treated during my first year out of physical therapy school is a great example of how powerful a tool the mind is in affecting our bodies. Iris was one of my first patients. Her diagnosis was intermittent cyanosis, which basically means that her extremities occasionally turned blue due to lack of oxygen.

Now, this isn't something we learn about in physical therapy school, so I took an extensive history that included a husband who had suffered a heart attack and been hospitalized a few months earlier. After this, Iris went home and scrubbed her house from top to bottom. The next morning she awoke with blue fingertips and lips. She went to see doctors, specialists, herbologists, acupuncturists—you name it. No one had a clue as to the solution, and neither did I.

I decided to do some range-of-motion and strength testing. As we began moving, her fingertips, toes, and lips turned blue. As a first year grad, I knew enough to know this wasn't good. So I gave her a few stretches, making sure she understood to stop if anything turned blue, and sent her home. After she left the office, I called the referring doctor.

"I just had Iris in here, and she turned blue during my exam," I began.

"Yes, we've seen that happen too," replied the doctor.

"Have you done blood tests to see whether there is a chemical cause for her symptoms since this seems to correlate to her cleaning episode?" I asked.

"We've run every test we can think of. Nothing abnormal shows up," replied the doctor.

"I've never seen this before," I said.

"Neither have we," said the doctor. "Just do your best. We have to exhaust all avenues, and she's been through just about everything and everyone."

After three days practicing stretches, Iris returned. "Still turning blue," she offered. She was visibly upset. In my mind, I believed there was no exercise I could offer her that would correct this problem. I went back to her history and we talked.

"Iris, your husband had a heart attack three months ago," I began. She nodded, looking concerned.

"How's he doing?"

"He's much better. He's just started a walking program." She brightened a little.

Then what I needed to say next came to me. I looked her straight in the eyes and said, "Iris, your husband isn't going to die." She blinked.

"And neither are you," I continued. She blinked again and let out a deep breath.

I felt I was onto the source of her problem and continued, "Have you ever spoken of this to a therapist, counselor, priest, or friend? Anyone who you can confide in?"

"No, I haven't," she said.

"Then your treatment is to do so within the next four days. I'll see you in a week," I finished.

She came back next week, arm-in-arm with her husband and looking radiant.

"I just wanted my husband to meet you," she said and smiled. "This is him," she told her husband.

"How are you feeling?" I asked hopefully.

"No symptoms at all! Look!" She did all her exercises with no signs of cyanosis.

"Amazing," I said.

"I spoke with a therapist, and I feel so much better! I can do anything!" she exclaimed.

"Yes, you can," I said. We spoke some more and then hugged goodbye.

This has always struck me as a dramatic example of the mind's influence over the body. I cannot explain how Iris's mind affected her blood flow the way it did, but the connection seemed clear. We read stories almost daily in the newspaper about similar phenomena—people holding on to their lives through sheer will after being trapped in an earthquake or becoming elite athletes after conquering a life-threatening illness. We've all read or heard about Eastern mystics able to control almost every aspect of their bodies through meditative practice. Tapping into your brain's power to control your muscles, monitor your habits, or feed your desire to become better will be a large part of you remaining pain free after identifying and fixing the physical issues causing your pain. If Iris can restrict blood flow to her extremities and then reverse it, then surely we can master the way we move and function, and thereby live pain free.

My experience tells me that no matter what diagnosis you have or what kind of accident you were in, the body must learn to move correctly in order for tissues to be pain free or to experience significant pain reduction. This book teaches you to assess your movement patterns and correct the most common issues preventing ideal movement.

THE POWER OF WILLPOWER

Some people make goals because they'd like to achieve an end—and some people make goals because they must achieve an end. The second group are the people who get the work done, and usually above and beyond what I've asked of them. This is embodied in Ernie's truly inspirational story. Ernie had a traumatic brain injury as a result of being hit by a drunk driver while he was in a bike race. This happened three years earlier, and Ernie wanted to ride in that race again to prove to himself that he could do it. He had been through so much with his rehab, return to work, and family issues. This was one last big hurdle he wanted to clear.

I met Ernie and liked him immediately. I didn't have much experience working with people with brain injuries, just my clinical rotation during physical therapy school. I knew that these people need to limit stimuli (bright lights, loud noises, strength challenges, balance, and so on) because their brains have difficulty filtering the information.

But Ernie had fire in his eyes, and I could see he was committed in spite of his obvious challenges with cognitive, balance, strength, and flexibility deficits. We began by working in a dim, quiet room with no distractions and rigged up a bike with exercise stretch tubes to get him comfortable sitting on a bike again and relearning how to balance himself. I gave him instructions in simple sentences with plenty of time in between for processing. Once we mastered those skills, we moved on to standing balance and strengthening, while learning how Ernie's brain responded to physical exertion and simultaneously receiving instructions. He made excellent progress while we tailored his program to his specific needs.

I had the idea to make a set of training wheels for his transition to the bike outside. I visited several bike shops and spoke to their mechanics about my situation; each one told me to forget it, saying that I'd never get a person with a brain injury to ride a bike because it would be too difficult. That just fired me up even more. "You don't know Ernie," I thought.

Finally, we decided that I'd hold on to the bike while he rode. Ernie was scared at first, and so was I. If a person with a brain injury hits his head, he is more susceptible than the rest of us to further injury. Until that point it was relatively safe, innocuous work with no chance of further injuring his brain. But to achieve Ernie's goal of riding in his race, we had to take some risks. He had worked hard, and it was time to take the next big step.

Ernie and I went out to the parking garage, and he mounted the bike. I held on and ran with him while he pedaled and found his balance. We continued this for many sessions: I gave Ernie instructions, Ernie responded, and both of us learned how far we could push the envelope with this whole new level of difficulty.

Until one day Ernie said, "Let go."

"Are you sure?" I asked, huffing.

"Yes, I can do it. Let go," he answered.

I did. And he did.

He rode like a dream for 10 minutes. Once I saw his telltale signs of mental fatigue it was time to get off. While I held the bike for Ernie to dismount, I looked into his eyes. He was exhilarated and had engaged with plenty of stimuli for the day. Neither of us said a word. The hard work was done—then it was just a matter of building up his endurance.

I had never been as proud of someone as I was of Ernie that day in the garage. He stared down his fears and setbacks and rose above them in spite of all the evidence that he should not have been able to do what he did. He was and is a real hero and inspires me to this day. By the way, he rode in that race and finished, three years after being hit on his bike with only the chin strap of his helmet left intact. There is no reason you cannot achieve similar greatness and pride in your own accomplishments. You just have to begin.

Ernie faced his demons and conquered them. In spite of everything working against him, he drew from his vast inner strength to do what no one else believed he could do. Fixing chronic pain is no different except with one caveat: instead of others not believing in you, it is usually you who does not believe in yourself. It's no wonder, after seeing specialists and therapists who couldn't help you or after seeing images of structural damage and being told this was the cause of your pain. This time will be different because you will have the keys to unlock the mysteries of your pain.

ATTENTION AND AWARENESS

Chronic aches and pains aren't just for those who have been involved in accidents. I've found similar biomechanical problems at the roots of chronic pain in people who have had traumatic accidents as well as in those who didn't. Therefore, I believe accidents expose and exacerbate existing vulnerabilities in our bodies. Fixing someone who was involved in a motor vehicle accident that resulted in chronic neck pain has been no different than helping someone who has had headaches and neck pain for decades and has never been involved in an accident. They both require an understanding of how poor function is feeding the problem and what needs to be corrected to eliminate pain. Essentially, in order to fix your body and eliminate chronic pain, you need to pay attention to how your body moves.

I used to work at a health club. While I was in the locker room changing after a workout one day, a man approached me.

"Hey, do you mind taking a look at my arm? I bumped it last week, and now I don't seem to have the strength I used to," he said.

"Sure," I said.

In three seconds, I knew exactly what his problem was; he had completely severed his biceps tendon at the elbow. His injured arm was visibly smaller than the other, and the biceps muscle was curled up in a little ball up by his shoulder, similar to the way blinds roll up on a window. It was as if someone had stuffed a sock into his upper arm.

"You've ruptured your biceps tendon," I s&
to get an orthopedic surgeon to operate on it im&

He returned a few days later. "I saw a surge
wasn't torn," he said.

"Go see another surgeon—it's torn. I guara   ...d.
"And do it fast!" I added.

I saw him a month later in the locker room. "You were right,"
he said. "I saw another surgeon, and I had an emergency opera-
tion that day."

This man was not in touch with his body. Many of you reading this book are in a similar situation—not ever considering
how different parts of your body work together to create pain-
free movement. In the above case, a man had suffered a traumatic
blow to his arm that caused
his problem. In this regard, it
was a clear-cut issue that had
an easily pinpointed cause.
Chronic pain that isn't due to
trauma is often caused by a
gradual decline in the quality of the body's movements.

> If you are interested in learning
> more about specific neck
> diagnoses, go to the WebMD
> website (www.webmd.com) or
> the Family Doctor website (www.
> familydoctor.org). Both are good
> sources of medical information.

It is time for you to pay attention to your body, and my sincerest
hope is that the information in this book will help you do that. The
exercises in this book will help you if you check in with yourself
and become aware of your body. Always go back to your form
and think about what you are doing. Be present and be attentive—
you will be rewarded for it!

PAIN: THE GOOD AND THE BAD

The last item I'd like to address is pain avoidance. It is a natural reaction to avoid a stimulus that is hurting you. The operative
premise here is that it is hurting you. Quite often I need to educate
my clients regarding "good" pain versus "bad" pain. The discomfort of a fatigued muscle feels different than the pain of a muscle
strain or **impinged** joint—pain that indicates injury. Learning to

the difference between "good" pain (the temporary discomfort of retraining your body), and "bad" pain (pain that indicates injury) is important to your healing process.

Generally, what I'm referring to as "good" pain is a feeling of fatigue in the muscles or tissues you are exercising or trying to restore range of motion to. Muscle fatigue may be uncomfortable, but it doesn't mean that what we're doing is hurting us—in fact, that feeling of fatigue lets us know that we are getting stronger. Muscle fatigue also indicates that your body has had enough for the time being. Listen to your body. Stop when you need to. Don't try to push through another set of repetitions or add more weight until your body is ready. Avoiding the message your body is sending doesn't do you any favors and ultimately slows down your progress because ignoring good pain establishes compensatory behavior that can contribute to bad pain.

For example, imagine that you are performing a biceps curl, bending your elbow to bring your hand to the top of your shoulder and then lowering it back down to your side. Weight lifters perform this exercise with weights in their hands to strengthen the biceps muscles in the front of their arms. To maintain good form during this exercise, the arm should stay roughly at the midpoint of the trunk while curling the hand up and down. This helps the head of the arm bone, nestled in the shoulder socket, remain in its proper position with limited stress to the shoulder joint tissues.

Keeping the arm in a mechanically correct position fatigues the biceps muscles more quickly and with lighter weight. However, pushing past fatigue in order to reach a predetermined number of repetitions or lift heavier weight will force the elbow to compensate by rocking forward and back. When the elbow moves back, the head of the arm bone at the shoulder joint moves forward, often pulling the shoulder blade with it or stressing the tissues in the front of the shoulder. Over time this can create a host of mechanical problems in the shoulder joint.

Biceps fatigue during curls is good pain because it indicates that the muscle is being stimulated to strengthen and grow. This is what we are shooting for when performing the strengthening exercises at the end of this book. We want muscle stimulation and therefore improved strength and control of the bone or joint in question. In the biceps curl example, ignoring this fatigue to squeeze out a few more reps or allow you to lift more weight can cause shoulder joint problems. Become comfortable with and even rejoice in the fact that the muscle you are targeting is fatiguing. It is better to strengthen the muscle group incrementally rather than compensate your form—and your healing process—to squeeze out a few more repetitions. This is where bad pain comes in.

Avoidance of good pain—ignoring your body's signals—often leads to "bad" pain. Bad pain is more difficult to describe because everyone experiences it differently. It can be sharp or dull, nagging or acute. It is the pain you are trying to eliminate, the pain of injury or dysfunction. It is something you feel that you instinctively know shouldn't be happening.

You should only feel fatigue in the muscles you are targeting. Using the biceps curl example, if you feel pain at the shoulder or elbow joints while performing the curl, then you know you're experiencing bad pain. The biceps muscles are located between the shoulder and elbow joints. If you feel pain above or below the biceps muscles, it is likely that you are lifting too heavy a load or allowing your elbows to move too much. The habits that cause bad pain ultimately compromise your efforts, leading to tissue vulnerability and weakness—and more pain.

So often, clients are disappointed to find that they fatigue quickly when exercising with correct form. I happily point out that this is great news because they are finally activating and strengthening the right muscles without exacerbating their condition! Keep this in mind as you strengthen through your injury.

2 UNDERSTANDING YOUR ANATOMY

KNOWLEDGE *of any kind gets metabolized spontaneously and brings about a* CHANGE *in* AWARENESS *from where it is possible to create* NEW REALITIES.

—DEEPAK CHOPRA

Regardless of whether chronic pain has slowly crept into your life or it stems from a traumatic event such as a car accident, neck pain and headaches have their roots in two problems: poor shoulder function and poor neck function. Fixing problems in these two areas is fundamental to regaining control of your headaches and neck pain. If you also have shoulder pain and/or elbow pain, read *Fixing You: Shoulder & Elbow Pain*, as the shoulder is integral in fixing all these injuries. This book will cover most shoulder issues relating to neck pain.

I typically see problems such as **disk bulges**, **degenerative disk disease**, **disk herniations**, and arthritis in the neck—you name it. I call these **structural diagnoses** because they describe a physical problem that can be seen on an MRI or other scan. Because these physical problems can be seen with a scan, the conclusion is that the structural damage is the cause of your pain. I liken this to seeing an X-ray of a broken left thumb and appropriately casting it to heal without realizing that the right hand is continually hitting it with a hammer. Until we can make the right hand stop, the left thumb will continue to be reinjured, if it ever really heals at all. Yes, the broken bone is painful, but the right hand continues to deliver more pain and injury, preventing true healing from occurring. I believe something similar is happening that causes these structural changes in the body. I interpret the presence of these structural diagnoses as evidence of **functional problems**.

Functional problems are those in which muscles or joints do not move optimally, creating stress to the tissues. In my experience, functional problems lead to structural diagnoses and pain. This may occur due to faulty movement patterns, weakness, limited range of motion, old injuries, or all of these factors. I believe the repeated stress from functional problems leads to physical changes in the body such as degenerative disks, arthritis, or disk bulges—in other words, structural diagnoses. Structural diagnoses do not describe the roots of the pain but are instead symptoms the root problems create. If you have these diagnoses, do not despair! You can be helped!

But here's the interesting thing: Pain can be eliminated even though the structural diagnosis remains. Almost all my clients who come to me with a structural diagnosis have become pain free or have at least significantly reduced their pain. This happens because we target the functional problems, not the structural diagnosis. Having said that, almost all neck pain and headaches I treat are primarily due to poor shoulder blade (**scapula**) function—regardless of the structural diagnosis involved. In the following pages you will read stories of people who suffered for years with neck pain—which vanished once the shoulder blade was corrected. Correcting scapular problems will be the foundation of your approach to fixing your neck pain or headaches.

The good news is it is easier than you might imagine. While there are many parts to the equation, after reviewing the mechanics more closely, you will understand the simplicity of the underlying order and precision in neck function. Learning about the fundamentals of neck and shoulder function will help you visualize exactly how they should be working throughout the day. When we are finished, you will have a complete understanding of the whys and hows behind your pain and how to fix them.

You might ask, "Why should I take the time to learn about the anatomy of neck and shoulder function when I can just do the exercises?" I promise I will make learning this as painless and interesting as possible—the last thing I want to be is another pain in the neck! But remember, a large part of healing yourself is visualizing ideal movement as well as knowing where you are going wrong. Your current habits, weaknesses, or deficits in range of motion are causing your pain. It will require your attention to your body to fix these problems. In order to remain pain free, you will need to be able to visualize optimal shoulder and neck function and check your own mechanics against that visualization. If you have little or no interest in understanding the whys and hows behind your neck pain, you can skip to Section 3: Corrective Exercises to get started on your program, but I don't recommend this. While these exercises will reduce or eliminate your pain, altering your habits will keep you pain free.

THE ROOTS OF NECK PAIN & HEADACHES

Understanding proper shoulder mechanics—how your shoulder muscles work and affect your head and neck—is fundamental to eliminating neck and pain and headaches. Looking at a skeleton (Figure 2.1), you'll see that the bones are stacked on top of each other at almost every joint. Joint compression due to gravity is one factor that helps your body stay in alignment. But look more closely at the shoulder and you'll see that its only connection to the rest of the skeleton is via the horizontal collarbone at the front of the rib cage. This joint acts as something of a fulcrum for shoulder function. The rest is just floating in space.

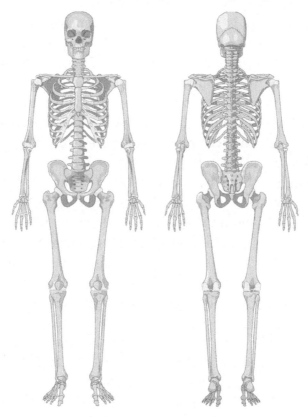

The Human Skeleton

Figure 2.1 The human skeleton is largely comprised of bones stacked on top of each other. This allows gravity and compression to assist with stabilization and tracking of joints. In contrast, the shoulder uses muscle, tendon, and ligaments to hold it in position. This creates a paradox between stabilization and mobilization.

How can that tiny **clavicle** hold up the shoulder? It can't. What holds the shoulder in position is not joint compression, but muscle tone—specifically the trapezius, **levator scapula, serratus anterior,** and **rhomboid muscles,** as well as ligaments (Figure 2.2). Two of these muscles, the levator scapula and the trapezius, also attach to the neck bones (**cervical spine**) and/or base of the skull. Because the shoulder joint is held in position by muscle tone rather than by joint compression, and some of these muscles attach to the neck and head, unnatural shoulder mechanics—a functional problem—can cause neck pain and headaches.

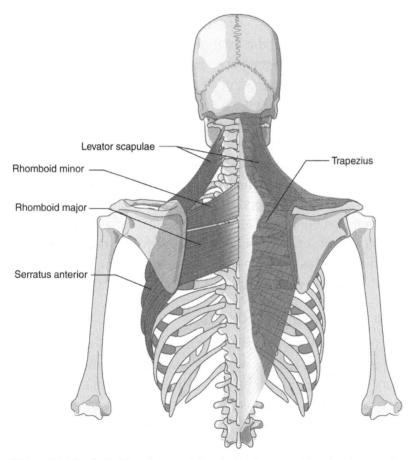

Figure 2.2 Muscles holding the scapula in correct alignment. Note that the trapezius and levator scapulae attach to the head and neck. The levator scapulae lie deep in relation to the trapezius and are often overworked in individuals with upper trapezius weakness or whose upper trapezius is overly lengthened.

The upper portion of the trapezius muscle helps elevate the scapula both at rest and in overhead positions. Often the upper trapezius will become weak or long, allowing the shoulder blade to sink too far down on the trunk. This leaves the levator scapula vulnerable because it then must do the work of two muscles. The levator scapula attaches from the scapula to the upper four **vertebrae** of the neck. When

> The **levator scapula** muscle is where most people typically feel neck pain. This is because the levator scapula often becomes overloaded due to poor function of other key muscles.

repeatedly tugged on, this muscle contributes to neck extension, rotation, and/or compression—especially when the deep neck- stabilizing muscles (located in the front of the neck) are weaker than the adverse forces acting on the neck. This can occur asymmetrically, creating compression, rotation, or extension on one side of the neck more than on the other. When the neck is unable to stabilize against these forces, neck pain or headaches result.

Now think about how heavy your arm is, including your shoulder blade. Think of all the muscles, bones, nerves, blood, tendons, and ligaments. How heavy do you think all that may be? Ten pounds? Fifteen? Twenty? If the muscles holding your arm in place—your shoulder muscles—aren't functioning properly, suddenly you've got a big pendulum hanging from your neck, dragging it around. This can contribute to compression, rotation, and extension of the **cervical vertebrae**, as well as disk problems.

PROPER SHOULDER MECHANICS

One of the biggest keys to neck function is a shoulder blade that works properly. The scapula needs to rest and move in a fairly precise way in order to unload the neck and shoulder joints.

One of the scapula's functions is to support arm movements in overhead positions by rotating, elevating, and sliding out underneath the arm as it reaches up. It becomes the foundation on which arm function rests. If that isn't happening, the shoulder joint and neck are in for some real work. This eventually taxes the shoulder joint and neck and leads to neck pain, headaches, and other issues.

I use the term **depressed shoulder** to encompass a cluster of problems with the shoulder blade that usually come with shoulder blade depression and can cause chronic neck pain and headaches. The figure below shows you how the vertebrae are numbered and depicts

> When the scapula sits too low on the trunk, the shoulders are said to be depressed. Usually this is due to lengthened or weakened **upper trapezius** muscles. When a shoulder blade is depressed, several other problems typically also exist.

how a normal and a depressed shoulder look at rest and overhead (Figure 2.3). In both pictures, the left shoulder is in a normal position and the right shoulder is depressed. Chances are that if a shoulder is sitting too low in a resting position, it will not elevate properly during overhead motions. This places strain on the neck because our friend, the levator scapula, is left to do more than its fair share of the work and transmits this stress to the cervical vertebrae.

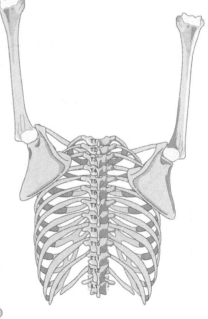

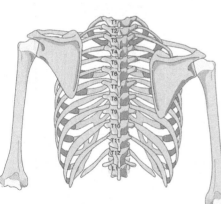

Depressed Right Scapula Resting   **Depressed Right Scapula Overhead**

Figure 2.3 Ideal and depressed scapulae in resting and overhead positions. The left resting scapula is normal, and the right side is depressed. You can see that the depressed scapula has limited elevation in the overhead position, creating strain on the neck by virtue of its muscle attachments.

The client's pictures depict what a depressed shoulder can look like in real life (Figure 2.4). In the front view, notice that the collar bones are horizontal. Ideally, they should angle upward as your eye travels away from the center of the chest and toward the shoulder. In the second picture from behind, we see how low the shoulder blades are in relation to the second **thoracic vertebra** (marked). You can also see the severe slope of her neck and shoulders, indicative of depressed shoulder blades. In the third picture, with her arms overhead, the scapulae have not rotated fully. You can see the angle her scapula achieves is closer to 30 degrees rather than the optimal 60 degrees of rotation needed to support the arm in overhead positions (see Landmarks and Solutions for Proper Shoulder Function, p. 44). Additionally, her shoulder blades are not adequately sliding away from her spine (**abducting**), also contributing to her shoulder blade dysfunction and, therefore, her neck pain.

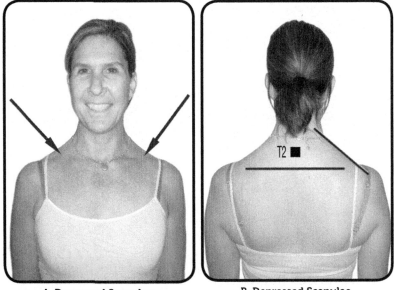

A. Depressed Scapulae,
Front View

B. Depressed Scapulae,
Back View

Figure 2.4 A Front view of a woman with depressed shoulder blades. Her collarbones are horizontal when they should be angled up toward the outside of the shoulder. **B** From the back, the scapulae sit far below the desired T2 or T3 position (marked). Also note the sharply sloped angle from the shoulder to the head.

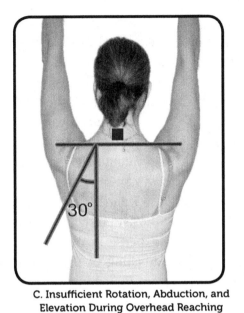

C. Insufficient Rotation, Abduction, and
Elevation During Overhead Reaching

Figure 2.4 C In overhead reaching, the shoulder blades rotate, abduct, and elevate
inadequately, increasing strain to the muscles connecting from the scapulae to the neck.

The body is designed to accept strain by dispersing it to adjacent structures. When one system does not properly accept strain, as in the case of a poorly functioning shoulder blade, strain is passed on to adjacent structures—in this case, the levator scapula and the cervical vertebrae. The neck, often sensitive to adverse stresses and weakened from poor posture, is unable to counter these constant forces. The vertebrae move when they should be stabilized, and neck pain results.

Although these deficits can exist irrespective of profession, lifestyle, or age there are a few behaviors that contribute to these functional problems. For instance, people who have been involved in extensive dance, yoga, or **Pilates** training or who have sedentary jobs that require long hours typing on computers often develop these issues. The reason dancers

> **While sitting at your desk** during the day, place a folded towel under your arm to **prop up your elbow**. This elevates your shoulder blade, unloading strain on the muscles connecting to your neck. Do this until your **upper trapezius muscle** is adequately retrained.

and yoga and Pilates practitioners develop these issues is that these disciplines strive for an aesthetic ideal of long, graceful necks. Although a long neck may look nice, it is not ideal for pain-free neck function. That is because to obtain the long neck, the shoulders must depress, which alters ideal shoulder mechanics and, therefore, neck function. Often it is taught that depressing the shoulders will strengthen the lower fibers of the trapezius muscle. This may activate those muscles but comes at the greater expense of overall shoulder function.

> **Do the Hand On Head exercise** anytime you experience pain to help eliminate neck pain and headaches while retraining your scapula to elevate properly.

Instead, the Trapezius Strengthening or the lift-off portion of the Arm Slide on the Wall exercises in Section 3: Corrective Exercises are more appropriate.

Gravity is the biggest culprit at sedentary jobs that require a lot of computer work. Because the arms are rarely elevated, gravity gradually pulls down the shoulder blades, causing tension at the levator scapula muscle. This will manifest as neck pain or headaches, and it could produce excessive stresses at the vertebrae themselves, resulting in structural diagnoses such as disk bulges, degenerated disks, and so on.

For women, there are two issues that particularly contribute to shoulder and therefore neck problems. The first is an ill-fitting bra with straps that loop over the outer shoulder or where the collar bone meets the scapula. To understand how this affects scapular positioning, hold your arm out to your side at shoulder height with a five-pound weight in your hand. With your arm still stretched out to the side, now put the five-pound weight on your shoulder. You'll notice it is far easier to hold the weight up when it is at the shoulder than when it is in your outstretched hand. This is because when trying to hold something up (the weight in this case), the further it is from the body means the harder it will be to hold up. The closer it is to your center, the easier it will be to hold up.

Bra straps that loop over the outer shoulder rather than closer to the neck have the same effect on the scapula: they drag it down over time because they pass over the outer shoulder rather than closer to the center. This is especially a problem for women with large breasts. I've seen bra straps that severely dig into the shoulder from the weight they carry, pulling the shoulder blades downward. Wide straps that pass closer to the neck or cross in the back can unburden the shoulder and help alleviate neck pain or headaches. Some department stores have personnel who specialize in fitting bras. When working with someone, be sure to mention your neck pain or headaches and the need to unload the shoulder blade as much as possible. Bringing in this book may help illustrate your needs.

The second problem particular to women is carrying a heavy bag or purse over one shoulder, dragging the shoulder down and stressing the muscles that attach from the shoulder blade to the neck. Some solutions for this include periodically switching the bag from one shoulder to the other, using bags that have double straps that disperse the weight (as in a backpack)—or simply cleaning out your bag to reduce the load.

Client Connection: Debbie's Depressed Shoulder

My deeper understanding of anatomy and biomechanics was triggered, in part, by working with one particular client, Debbie. Debbie came to me after suffering for 15 years with neck pain, migraines, and headaches stemming from two automobile accidents that occurred within a couple months of each other. She had a toddler in tow, which compounded the pain she had been experiencing all these years. She was diagnosed with disk bulges and degenerated disks in the cervical spine. She had been to doctors, specialists, massage therapists, chiropractors, physical therapists, acupuncturists—you name it.

I began working with her neck the way I usually did—finding **trigger points** and releasing them, going deeper with each visit. After the third visit, Debbie said her neck was feeling better, so I decided to assess her tolerance by very gently mobi-

A **trigger point** is a hypersensitive point or nodule in muscle that, when pressed, can refer pain to a distant site.

lizing her left shoulder to reproduce some of the trauma she initially experienced 15 years ago. The next day, she called me to say she was in the worst pain she'd felt in months. I was shocked.

I couldn't get her out of my mind for the next three days. Why had mobilizing her shoulder hurt her neck? On the third day, I had an epiphany: It wasn't her neck that was injured, it was her shoulder! She just felt the pain in her neck. Again, this goes back to the anatomy. I had instantly visualized that the levator scapula connecting from the shoulder blade to the neck was causing the neck pain because it was under too much tension due to its position—sitting too low. Instead of feeling pain where the levator scapula attaches at the shoulder, she felt pain at her neck, the more vulnerable part of her anatomy. This is called referred pain. Referred pain is a phenomena whereby the site of irritation is not where pain is felt. Instead, pain is felt further from the site. For instance, in the case of a rotator cuff injury at the top of the shoulder, pain may be felt further down the arm or even in the elbow. Similarly, a hip joint injury may be felt as groin pain.

> Pain in the body often occurs at the most mobile joints. Imagine repeatedly bending a thin copper pipe. Eventually the pipe will break at the point where excessive motion occurs. It is the same in the body.

I convinced her to come in again for treatment (and believe me, this was no small feat after the pain I had put her in). When I told her it wasn't her neck but her shoulder that was the root of her problems, she looked at me sideways.

"But no one's ever looked at my shoulder before. Besides, my shoulder doesn't hurt. It's my neck that hurts," she said.

I'm sure she thought I was cuckoo, but I convinced her to let me have a closer look at her shoulder and told her that if I didn't help her, she need not come back again. Lo and behold, her shoulder blade did not look right. It sat too low (**depressed**) on her trunk by about one and a half inches and about an inch too far away from her spine (**abducted**). So I positioned it correctly and held it there with my hands.

"How's that?" I asked hopefully.

"My pain's gone," she said, surprised. She continued moving

her head around, exclaiming, "No pain!"

After at least 15 years of shoulder dysfunction, I assumed her muscles would not be able to hold the corrected position on their own. So I taped her shoulder into position and sent her on her way. After three days, she reported that her pain and headaches were significantly decreased.

The Fixing You Approach for a Depressed Shoulder

A poorly functioning shoulder blade that relentlessly tugged at her neck was at the root of Debbie's headaches and neck pain. Remember the levator scapula and the trapezius muscle that connect the shoulder to the neck? When those muscles aren't working properly, the shoulder blade doesn't move as it should, becoming dead weight hanging on the neck. In Debbie's case, I believe her two motor vehicle accidents 15 years earlier exposed existing vulnerabilities in her neck and shoulders. Although it is impossible to know for sure, I believe they were already depressed and abducted. They probably also didn't rotate or elevate well when the arm moved. But her muscles were just strong enough to function without pain.

The accident essentially stressed that weakened area and pushed the tissues' capacity to maintain shoulder function past their limits. The muscles could not heal because the trapezius muscle was stretched beyond its optimal length, and proper scapular dynamics were never restored. The bottom line is the tissues were never given a chance to rest due to the constant weight of the shoulder and arm tugging on them. In the absence of adequate help from the trapezius muscle, the levator scapula was asked to do more work. It is a thin muscle with limited capacity for carrying the load of the shoulder blade and arm, causing the pain that Debbie felt in her neck.

I believe Debbie had frequent migraines and headaches because this stress acted as a trigger to the nerves responsible for the headaches. When she became busy, she spent more time on the computer or running around carrying a bag on her shoulder, which depressed the shoulder more and triggered the headaches and migraines. She attributed this to stress, but it was actually the change in her activities and posture during stressful times that triggered her pain. Once we had identified the mechanical problem, we could isolate and work on the muscles that weren't working properly as well as the behaviors that led to her pain.

First, I taught Debbie how her scapula should move correctly and gave her the All-Fours Rocking Stretch exercise to practice. The better the scapula moves, the less tugging occurs on the neck. Then I taught Debbie how to activate her shoulder blade muscles to hold the shoulder blade in its correct position with Trapezius Strengthening and Arm Slides. Activating these muscles unloaded the scapula's dead weight from the neck.

Her pain almost instantly disappeared once we began this course of treatment. As you will learn, the interesting thing about all the exercises Debbie used is that not one of them directly involves working on the neck. Instead, all of them focus on correcting shoulder blade function. It will be the same with you as well. Yes, your neck posture may be a component that needs some help, but in my experience, correcting problems with the shoulder blade is 70 to 100 percent of fixing neck pain and headaches for the reasons outlined above.

LANDMARKS AND SOLUTIONS FOR PROPER SHOULDER FUNCTION

Assessing and correcting your shoulder blade will prove to be a powerful ally in fixing your neck pain. If the shoulder blade isn't sitting properly on the trunk at rest, it probably isn't working correctly when the arm is moving. There are five landmarks I look for in assessing shoulder blade function. The first two address how the shoulder blade is resting when the arm is down. In this situation, I like to see how low and far from the spine the shoulder blade is sitting. Then I observe how the scapula looks when the arm is reaching up. In particular, I'm interested in seeing if it has rotated, elevated, and slid out far enough to support the arm in the air. Remember, the shoulder blade is supposed to function as a foundation from which the arm moves and works when it is elevated. Restoring shoulder function to reach these ideal positions eliminates most neck pain and/or headaches.

In my experience, there is rarely just one deficient landmark.

Especially if a resting-position landmark is off, the stage is set for dysfunction when the arm moves. Restoring correct movement patterns can actually be a very quick process. I've had clients with only 30 degrees of scapular rotation reach 55 degrees in one session and eliminate their pain. The exercises outlined in this book are designed to correct these landmarks—and, therefore, shoulder and neck function.

Assessing your shoulder landmarks can be tricky, but it is important for understanding the big picture of shoulder function. You will need assistance to become aware of these landmarks as they are all found in the back of the shoulder. Referring to Figures 2.4, 2.5, and 2.6 may help you visualize the assessments. If only one shoulder is painful, it is often helpful to compare your pain-free shoulder to your troublesome shoulder's landmarks. However, this doesn't always work out because even the pain-free shoulder usually has some problems. I believe the reason you may experience pain in only one arm even though both exhibit similar deficits has to do with how you are using the injured arm. Most often, it is the arm that carries your briefcase or purse—anything that drags it down. Perhaps it is the arm that you do not lean on when sitting in a chair. Leaning on an elbow while sitting pushes the shoulder up and unloads irritated or weak tissues. If one arm is never weight bearing, it doesn't get this temporary benefit.

When assessing your shoulders, it is best to find a physical therapist to ensure that the correct assessment is made. However, if this is not possible, I've attempted to make it as straightforward as possible for someone to help you. You can find video clips of these assessments on the website at **www.FixingYou.net**. Just type in the code at the back of the book to access the video clips.

Landmark 1: Scapula resting at T2 or T3

The top of the shoulder blade should sit roughly at the second (T2) or third (T3) thoracic vertebra (Figure 2.5). I often see scapulae that are sitting lower than this. When this displacement occurs, the upper trapezius is typically too long and/or too weak to hold up the scapula. I see this problem in nearly everyone with neck pain.

Depressed shoulder blades can increase tension on the muscles connecting the scapulae to the neck, specifically the levator scapulae discussed above, and can lead to neck pain and headaches. It also sets the stage for inadequate elevation of the scapulae during overhead motions, further compromising those muscles and tissues.

Exercise Recommendations: The All-Fours Rocking Stretch, Arm Slides, and Hand on Head are useful exercises to help correct depressed shoulder blades. Other exercises could include Latissimus Dorsi Stretch and Side-lying Arm Slides.

Daily Tip: Try this simple movement to train your upper trapezius to work better: Shrug your shoulder up as your arm reaches overhead and allow it to remain up while the arm lowers. When sitting, prop your elbows up so the shoulders sit higher than normal. To achieve this, you can change your work chair, or rest your elbows on a folded towel at your desk to help elevate the shoulders and reduce stress to the neck.

Landmark 2: Scapula border 3 inches from the spine

The **vertebral border** of the scapula (the border that is closest to and runs roughly parallel to the spine) needs to be approximately three inches from the spine (Figure 2.5). This is true whether you're five feet tall or seven feet tall. I see problems in both directions—either too close to the spine (adducted) or too far away (abducted)—but usually they sit too far away from the spine. People with abducted shoulder blades that rest too far from the spine may have rounded shoulders or arms that are rotated inward. People with adducted shoulder blades that rest too close to the spine typically have a more erect posture because they are pinching the shoulder blades together.

Exercise Recommendations: The Trapezius Strengthening exercise is helpful to correct an abducted scapula. Also, when performing Arm Slides or the All-Fours Rocking Stretch, squeeze your shoulder blades together to begin in a corrected position three inches from the spine. Correcting an adducted scapula is simple—just relax the shoulder blade so it slides out to the ideal three-inch position.

Daily Tip: Monitor your shoulders during the day, and learn to detect when they are becoming too rounded or too close together. Because it can be difficult to get a sense of where your shoulder blades are in relation to your spine, have a friend check you periodically to see if you are on target. If your shoulders are too far from your spine, initially you will feel that you must work hard to squeeze them in. If they are too close to your spine, at first you will feel that you are slouching when you correct them. Again, have a friend check to make sure you've got it right. Be sure your head does not move forward while you are adjusting! It will take just a little time to learn how to find the ideal three-inch position, but you will master it quickly.

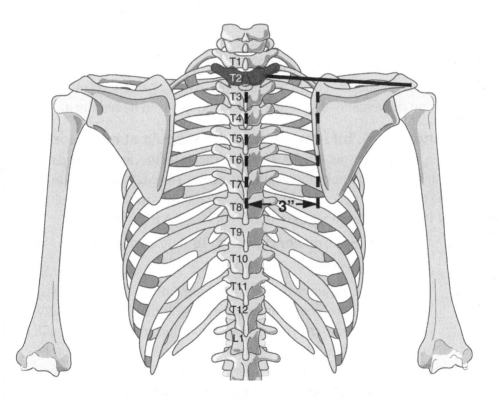

Landmarks for Resting Shoulder Position

Figure 2.5 A shoulder at rest should have its vertebral border approximately three inches from the spine. The top of the scapula should align with T2 or T3.

Landmark 3: Scapular rotation at 60 degrees

The shoulder blade needs to rotate outward about 60 degrees when the arm is in an overhead position (Figure 2.6). I often see scapulae with only 30 to 45 degrees of rotation. Limited rotation means the arm is not supported adequately when moving in overhead positions, and this can lead to neck pain.

Exercise Recommendations: To help correct inadequate scapular rotation, do the All-Fours Rocking Stretch and Arm Slides.

Daily Tip: When raising your arm, visualize reaching up with the shoulder blade instead of the hand. You will get the same result—your hand being overhead—but it will feel completely different. This is because you are using the scapular muscles to help lift your arm rather than letting your shoulder muscles do all the work. This will help mobilize the scapula, better activating key muscles that have been lying dormant. Again, initially this movement will feel awkward or unnatural to you. This is because your movement habits have created a perception of "natural movement" that is inaccurate and needs to be retrained.

Landmark 4: Inferior angle of the scapula at mid-thorax

The bottom corner of the scapula, the **inferior angle**, needs to reach approximately the midpoint of the rib cage on the side of the trunk (Figure 2.6). I frequently see the inferior angle fall short of this mark, reaching only to the back of the rib cage.

Exercise Recommendations: To help correct this, do the All-Fours Rocking Stretch and Arm Slides.

Daily Tip: Again, visualize reaching up with your shoulder blade instead of your hand when reaching overhead. Typically, if you can improve your scapular rotation, the abduction will come along too. That is because we measure the abduction by where the bottom corner (inferior angle) of the scapula moves. If the shoulderblade is rotating correctly, that means the inferior angle is swinging out to the side of the trunk in the correct position as well.

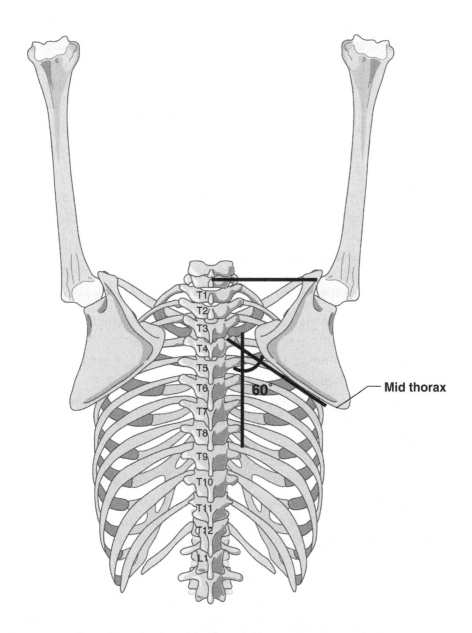

Landmarks for Overhead Shoulder Position

Figure 2.6 In the overhead position, the scapula should ideally rotate 60 degrees, elevate to approximately C7, and abduct to the mid trunk (mid thorax).

Landmark 5: Scapular elevation to C7

The upper, outer edge of the scapula needs to elevate to approximately the seventh cervical vertebra (C7; see Figure 2.6). Especially when the scapula is depressed to begin with, the chances of reaching C7 are much reduced. When the scapula does not elevate properly, increased stress is placed on the muscles attaching the scapula to the neck and head, potentially causing spinal compression or rotation. This is often at the root of neck pain and/or headaches.

> **Exercise Recommendations:** The All-Fours Rocking Stretch, Arm Slides, and Hand on Head are useful exercises to help correct scapular elevation.

> **Daily Tip:** To train your upper trapezius to work better, shrug your shoulder up as your arm reaches overhead, and allow it to remain up while your arm lowers. Visualize reaching up with your scapula instead of just with your hand.

HEADACHES: THE NECK & SHOULDER CORRELATION

The information above addresses shoulder biomechanics and how and why they contribute to neck pain and headaches. So let's talk briefly about common habits more specific to the neck that also factor into neck problems and headaches.

The most common type of neck problem stems from holding your neck in extension, such as happens with a forward-head position, in which the head sits too far forward on the trunk. Most if not all our activities during the day involve maintaining or increasing our neck's extension. The head moves forward (increases neck extension) during a variety of activities such as driving, working on a computer, or raising and lowering an arm. Ideally, your head should sit over your shoulders, not in front of them. When the head moves forward, it places the cervical spine in extension—especially at the base of the skull. The muscles at the back of the head that connect the base of the skull to the neck shorten to accommodate this position. Typically, in the clients I've worked with, headaches are commonly caused by these muscles being excessively shortened or strained. Correcting a for-

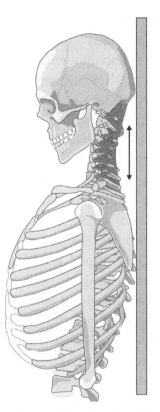

Proper Head Alignment

Figure 2.7 When correcting your head's position, focus on lengthening the muscles at the base of your skull.

ward-head position can restore the muscles to their proper lengths and decrease chronic headaches (Figure 2.7).

Learning which behaviors trigger the head to move forward and either modifying those behaviors or your neck's response to them is important to completely fixing neck pain or headaches. Throughout the day, monitor your neck and correct excessive forward-head or extended-neck positions. I've found the best way to do this is to set up a system of reminders such as stickers on the computer, phone, clock, dashboard of your car—anything you look at frequently. Wear a special bracelet or ring or your watch on the opposite wrist to remind you to periodically check in on your head and neck position.

One of my clients, the CEO of a large advertising firm, invited me over for a dinner party once. I noticed that her head moved forward every time she engaged in conversation. I pointed this out to her during our next appointment, and she has been working to break this habit since. Now, whenever she experiences neck pain at luncheons or meetings, she is able to check in with herself and use the simple technique of lengthening the muscles at the base of her skull. I have yet to be invited back for a party though—I hope she didn't think I was nagging!

Driving is an activity that can really pull your neck forward. This is because it can be a fairly stressful activity depending on road conditions, traffic, and the demands of your schedule. Put a sticker on the dashboard to help you remember to stay calm and check in on your neck posture. Every time you see that sticker, you can do a quick check of your neck position and fix it by lengthening the muscles at the base of your skull.

If you work out at a gym, you have probably noticed that the TVs are up high on the walls. You must look up to watch them, which promotes excessive neck extension. Simply don't do this. Find something else to occupy your mind for the 20 or 60 minutes while you are training. Once your neck pain or headache issue has resolved, you can go back to watching TV, but for the time being, focus on eliminating all the habits in your life that feed your pain.

Client Connection: Helen's Headaches

Helen was a fortysomething executive in an energy firm. She had a 20-year history of headaches and had been around the medical block in search of solutions. She had been diagnosed with degenerative disk disease in four of her cervical vertebrae. I had previously worked with her personal trainer who referred her to me because they were not able to progress her arm strengthening without causing neck pain and headaches. What I found was not so different than Debbie's case: a shoulder blade that sat too low and out to the side.

However, Helen also held her head in an extended, or forward-head, position. This posture caused shortening in the muscles at the back of her head that attach her neck to the base of her skull. These muscles are often closely correlated with headaches. Pressing on the muscles at the base of the skull will often reproduce headaches. Maintaining this pressure will usually take the headache away. My experience has shown that by eliminating or reducing stresses acting on these muscles, headaches are reduced or eliminated for good.

What's more, it is common for people to carry their head slightly side-bent or rotated due to their work station setup, their daily habits, or muscle tightness. If the head is habitually side-bent or rotated, asymmetrical pressure can be placed on these muscles, causing headaches on one side of the head versus the other. This was the case with Helen.

The Fixing You Approach for a Forward Head

I gave Helen the same exercises I gave Debbie, with a few additions. Observing Helen's movement patterns showed me that whenever her arm moved overhead, her head and neck moved further into extension. So while performing the All-Fours Rocking Stretch exercise, we made sure that she lengthened the back of her neck in order to avoid compressing the spine. It took quite a bit of work for her to get this right as her habits were so deeply ingrained. But she stayed with it because her neck pain was almost eliminated after performing just a few repetitions of these exercises.

I gave Helen the Neck Extensor Stretch to elongate the muscles at the base of her skull and to activate the muscles in the front of her neck to help hold her head in a better position. I also began Helen's strengthening program with Arm Slides to retrain her shoulder blade to work correctly. It was important that she learn to move her arm overhead without allowing the neck to extend or compress the vertebrae, so the cue I gave her was to continually lengthen the base of the skull while performing the exercises.

Sleep habits can also contribute to neck pain, as it did in Helen's case. After observing her posture while lying on her side, we saw that one of her shoulders excessively slid away from her spine (abducted). This caused her neck to move into slight extension again and was painful. On her second visit, she was able to perform her other exercises correctly, and her neck pain and headaches were dramatically reduced. Therefore, I felt it was safe to introduce the

Trapezius Strengthening exercise. I taught her how to squeeze her shoulder blades together and she performed five repetitions. I then retested her side-lying sleeping position to note the effects on her neck pain. It was all but gone after only one set of the exercises! She had to continue the strengthening until she developed proper tone in her trapezius muscles, but we both had a good feeling that this was exactly what she needed to help her with sleeping. This ended up being her last visit. She had all the tools necessary to prevent or eliminate her headaches.

I had another client who had worked hard to correct many of the movement dysfunctions we had discovered that led to her neck pain, yet the pain returned. I was baffled until I asked her how she slept. She told me she slept on her stomach. This is a bad position for the neck because it is forced into severe rotation for prolonged periods of time. Not only did she sleep on her stomach, but she did so with a pillow under her head. So now we added extreme neck extension together with the rotation to her troubles. No wonder she couldn't get better! If you sleep on your stomach, stop! This is probably the worst position for your neck and back.

> When you lie on your side, your top shoulder and arm will drop to the bed, pulling your shoulder blade forward and creating an extension stress in the cervical spine. To prevent this, try sleeping with your arm resting on a pillow to help your shoulder blade remain in an optimal position.

Sleeping on your back can also be bad—especially with a thick pillow under your head. The pillow essentially holds the head in a forward position and allows the muscles attaching from the neck to the base of the skull to remain short. This reinforces the forward-head position when you are standing and creates a vicious cycle wherein the head is not permitted to return to an ideal position.

Some of my clients have had great success in diminishing their neck pain and headaches by reducing the thickness of the pillows they sleep on. If you are planning to try this, start by making

> Sleep with a body pillow to help support your arms or legs comfortably.

small changes, and let them take effect over a period of a couple weeks before further lowering the pillow's profile. Not all people will tolerate sleeping with a lower pillow, and it could make matters worse if too much change is attempted all at once. It may take several weeks or months to tolerate a thinner pillow that doesn't support the head in an extended-neck position.

> **Stick with changing your habits,** and eventually you will become comfortable sleeping in a position other than on your stomach.

Likewise, if you sleep on your stomach, try falling asleep on your side or back instead. Gradually this will not feel so foreign. If you wake up in the middle of the night to use the bathroom, return to your back or side. Give yourself some time. Making abrupt changes during sleep can irritate the neck. You are sleeping for six to eight hours, which is a significant period of time to maintain a drastic change in your accustomed sleeping position. Be easy on yourself. Remember, the goal is to lengthen the muscles attaching the base of the skull to the neck.

For many, correcting a forward-head position by performing the Neck Extensor Stretch and through monitoring habits will yield great returns. For example, how you sit in a chair can dramatically effect neck pain, either reducing it or feeding it (Figure 2.8). I often ask clients to put timers on their desks or attached to their belts and set them to go off every half hour, reminding them to

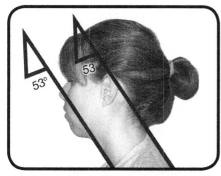
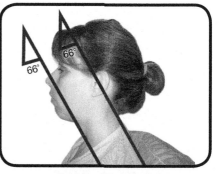

A. Normal Sitting Posture   **B. Using Chair Back**

Figure 2.8 A This woman has a forward head while sitting. Note the angle of her neck. **B** Resting against the back of the chair reduces her forward-head posture and her neck pain.

check in on their neck posture. Doing this for a week or two will yield faster relief from headaches because you are constantly correcting your painful habits.

For those on their feet, I ask them to put their backs against the wall, feet out from the wall, and bend their knees until they can comfortably rest their head against the wall. From here, I ask them to lengthen the base of the skull. Then, I ask them to raise their arms for two repetitions, keeping the neck long in the back. When they slide back up and resume their work, their neck pain has been reduced—and good habits have been reinforced.

Fixing your habits that lead to neck pain will require attention on your part and perhaps a friend or therapist to help you get the exercises exactly right, but you can do it!

Fixing a Forward Head

Correcting a forward head is trickier than you might think. Most people bring the head into further extension when trying to correct their heads' position. Instead, visualize gently lengthening the back of the head to correct it (Figure 2.9). An easy way to do this is to place your finger at the base of your skull in the back and help it lengthen toward the ceiling. You might notice that your chin nods slightly to your chest to achieve this—perfect! The axis of the nod should be at the base of your skull instead of further down the neck. You are activating the deeper muscles in the front of your neck (neck flexors), which are most likely weak or long. Keep your focus on elongating the muscles at the base of the skull instead of nodding the chin, as the latter can result in improper movements of the neck. Be gentle! You've had years to develop your forward head; it won't be fixed in a day.

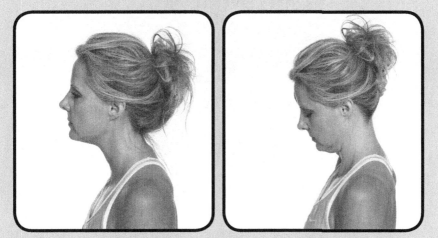

Figure 2.9 Correcting a forward head (left) involves lengthening the muscles at the base of the skull in the back of the neck (right).

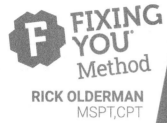

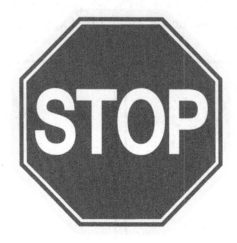

3 | CORRECTIVE EXERCISES

I've been a few places like that where I've thought, "A BREAKTHROUGH *is possible here. This is the place for the* EXERCISES *that will bring me to* WHERE I WANT TO BE."*

—JOSEPH CAMPBELL

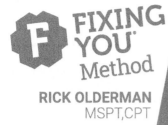
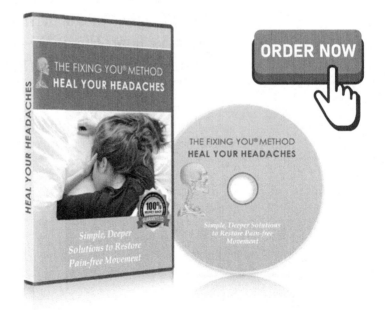

The following exercises are meant to develop your strength and improve your range of motion. If you find a particular exercise difficult, chances are it is because of weakness or movement dysfunction. Take that as a cue that you need help in that spot and therefore should practice it until you've mastered it. Any pain you experience performing the exercises should be considered bad pain, unless you are experiencing fatigue, which is good pain. If you experience real discomfort, stop immediately, carefully read the instructions or visit **www.FixingYou.net** to ensure you are performing the exercise correctly, and try again. It could be that you are simply trying too hard and need to relax. Many people try to completely fix range of motion issues in one day. Instead, take your time. The fact that your pain is diminishing will be proof that you are on the right track and it is just a matter of time before it is completely eliminated.

> **Resist the temptation** to push too far too fast, and remember to **listen to your body**. If you feel pain, stop!

Good form is critical, and you may need some help developing new habits. For instance, when performing the All-Fours Rocking Stretch exercise, your head will typically extend and your neck vertebrae will compress, resulting in your eyes looking forward or up while rocking backward onto your heels. Have a friend help you correct your form by visually monitoring your neck as you perform this exercise. They should make sure your neck remains long in the back.

> **Poor form or posture** during strength training can promote neck pain. Be sure your neck does not arch, which will create neck extension and feed your pain. **Keep the back of your neck long.**

An easy way to check this is to put the fingers of one hand at the base of the neck and the fingers from the other hand at the base of the skull. As you rock backward onto your heels, the distance between the fingers of both hands should not decrease. All of this is detailed in the All-Fours Rocking Stretch video clip online. You will not be aware of this in the beginning, and it will require some time for you to relearn how to maintain the long neck.

The same holds true for Arm Slides. As your arm slides up, your head will typically try to extend, side-bend, and/or rotate to one side. Resisting these motions will strengthen your weakened neck muscles and reinforce healthy movement patterns. Again, have a friend or therapist monitor this for you, so you can effectively learn new movement habits. If you find an exercise that feels good, then do it as often as you can. Your body knows what it likes—trust it! Restoring range of motion and getting things moving the way they should always helps healing and reduces pain. Videos of all the exercises can be viewed on my website at **www.FixingYou.net**. Just type in the code found in the back of this book.

During the first session or two, I typically begin with stretches such as the All-Fours Rocking Stretch or Neck Extensor Stretch. Stretching exercises are generally held for 30 to 60 seconds. Performing two to five repetitions is usually all that is needed to experience a positive effect. During the first week or two, I also typically ask my clients to commit to performing their stretches as often as possible (two to five times each day for two to five repetitions per session) to aggressively restore range of motion, correct poor habits and, of course, reduce their symptoms. In fact, I ask my clients to perform the All-Fours Rocking Stretch every time they experience pain because it is so effective. It should always feel good to perform the stretching exercises, so this really shouldn't be a hard sell. You should feel that your pain has decreased as a result. After the symptoms have abated, you can cut down on the frequency of stretching and find the ideal number of times needed to keep your pain at bay. I recommend at least doing them first thing in the morning and last thing before bed, as most people's neck pain is aggravated during sleep.

After the stretching phase, begin strengthening. Add one exercise at a time to focus on getting it right and to test whether your pain is made worse by a particular movement. If your pain worsens, then your technique is incorrect or it is not the right exercise for you. Pay attention to how you are performing the exercise. Read the instructions carefully, and watch the video clips on the Fixing You website. Once you are successfully performing one exercise, then add the next. Each time you add a new strengthening exercise, do not change anything else about your program. This way, if you experience pain, you can isolate which exercise may be the cause.

Strengthening exercises generally require five to ten repetitions for one to two sets or until fatigue or compensatory movements occur. For instance, when doing the Arm Slides exercise, your neck may begin to extend in order to help your arms slide up the wall; this is a compensatory movement. If this occurs, either stop the exercise, limit your range of motion, or try to do it without allowing the neck to extend. Don't let your ego urge you to add more weight if you cannot control it well.

This is where your attention really comes in. The strengthening exercises are meant to strengthen specific muscles and, of course, should be pain free. For example, when performing Arm Slides, we are generally targeting upper trapezius strength as well as promoting scapular rotation, elevation, and abduction. Therefore, if you feel fatigue in your shoulders or biceps or feel pain in your neck, then you should stop and pay attention to your form. The effort should be felt in the upper trapezius, between your shoulder and your neck—and you should not feel pain in your neck after the exercise because it is designed to eliminate pain, not trigger it. So take a moment to visualize the muscles you are attempting to train.

You may find that you must **temporarily decrease the weight** you are using. It's okay—fixing your neck is the **bigger picture.**

Another method that works well for my clients is to rapidly and briskly tap the muscle we are targeting. Sticking with the Arm Slides example, you can rapidly tap the upper trapezius muscle, located between your shoulder and your neck to "wake it up." Feel whether it has become harder due to its contraction. Keep tapping it to connect your consciousness to the muscle and develop your awareness of it and get it firing.

Just a little bit of strengthening will effect a positive change. As always, quality is more important than quantity. Strengthening exercises only need to be performed two to three times a day initially, although the Hand On Head exercise can be performed throughout the day to relieve symptoms and retrain the trapezius muscle. Once your pain diminishes and your habits are corrected, you may only need to perform the strengthening exercises once a day, once a week, once a month, or perhaps never again when your corrected movement habits are strengthening your muscles as needed, feeding your body rather than breaking it down.

The exercises below are the ones that I've found to provide almost immediate relief for most people. Begin with the stretches, focusing on improving your range of motion. Once you are performing them correctly, you can move on to the other three exercises

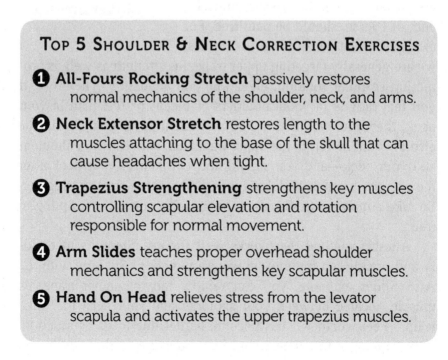

Top 5 Shoulder & Neck Correction Exercises

❶ **All-Fours Rocking Stretch** passively restores normal mechanics of the shoulder, neck, and arms.

❷ **Neck Extensor Stretch** restores length to the muscles attaching to the base of the skull that can cause headaches when tight.

❸ **Trapezius Strengthening** strengthens key muscles controlling scapular elevation and rotation responsible for normal movement.

❹ **Arm Slides** teaches proper overhead shoulder mechanics and strengthens key scapular muscles.

❺ **Hand On Head** relieves stress from the levator scapula and activates the upper trapezius muscles.

ALL-FOURS ROCKING STRETCH

This exercise passively restores normal shoulder joint and neck mechanics. It is a deceptively simple yet powerful exercise that yields big results.

THE FIXING YOU METHOD

Begin in a hands-and-knees position with your hands under your shoulders and your knees under your hips. Make sure your lower back is flat by drawing in your belly button. Also check that your neck is not arched in extension. If it is, then bring the chin down until you feel that your neck is relaxed and lengthened at the base of the skull. You will need someone to monitor this for you. Your eyes should be gazing directly below your nose, and you should maintain this position throughout the exercise.

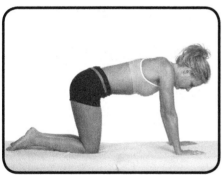 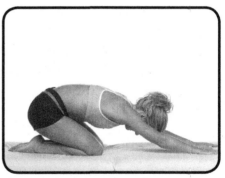

All-Fours Rocking Stretch,
start position

All-Fours Rocking Stretch,
end position

Exhale and rock back onto your feet. Feel that the floor is pulling your arms into an overhead position as shown in the picture. Allow your shoulders to be pulled into an overhead position while rocking backward. Initially it will feel like your shoulders are excessively shrugged up toward your ears; this is good because one of your problems may be shoulders that are sitting too low or are not elevating properly. Visualize the scapulae rotating out. Be sure the back of your neck remains lengthened (especially at the base of the skull) and the space between your ears and shoulders does not shorten or compress during the exercise. Return to the start position after holding for five breaths. Be sure your head maintains its long stretch and does not move back into extension while returning to the start position. Perform 2–5 repetitions.

COMMON ERRORS

- Rounding your upper back (thoracic spine) to assist moving your arms into an overhead position is not proper form. Keep the thoracic spine relaxed and flat.
- Your head remains up (extended) as you rock down to your feet. Instead, allow your chin to flex toward your chest, keeping your neck lengthened at the base of your skull. This can also serve to stretch the levator scapula.
- Trying to rock back too far may cause shoulder pain. Stop when you feel any pain.
- Don't rock back too rapidly before you are able to adequately control your neck. Slow down and understand what your neck and shoulders are doing at all times during the exercise.
- Maintain adequate shoulder elevation. Shrug your shoulders up when you initiate the rocking-back movement, or slide your hands forward prior to rocking back to help pull your shoulders up toward your ears.

NECK EXTENSOR STRETCH

This exercise improves range of motion in your neck and re-stores the neck-extensor muscles to their proper lengths. This is a particularly helpful exercise for those with a forward head. For those recovering from an acute injury of less than three months, be gentle when doing this exercise as it may stretch muscles too aggressively.

THE FIXING YOU METHOD
Lie on your back with your head resting comfortably. While slowly bringing your arms into an overhead position resting on the floor,

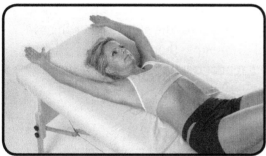
Neck Extensor Stretch

lengthen the back of your neck, separating the base of the skull from your neck; doing this properly will cause your chin to slight-ly nod toward the front of your neck.

Hold for 30–60 seconds, focusing on lengthening the base of the skull rather than tucking your chin. Bring your arms back down to your sides, making sure your neck does not arch. Maintain the lengthened position at the base of your skull. If this maneuver is diffi-cult, then practice it with a limited range of motion until you can con-trol your neck extension. Perform 2–5 repetitions.

COMMON ERRORS
- Focusing on nodding the chin forward rather than lengthen-ing the muscles in the back of the neck may activate a for-ward-head position.
- If your shoulder pain increases when your arms are overhead, rest your arms on pillows to find a comfortable position.
- Don't move your arms too rapidly before correcting neck extension. Move slowly to be sure you are performing the exercise correctly.

TRAPEZIUS STRENGTHENING

This exercise restores trapezius muscle strength to assist in shoulder elevation and scapular rotation.

THE FIXING YOU METHOD

Lie on your stomach. Place your hands on top of your head or behind your neck, fingers interlaced, with your elbows resting on the floor. If you cannot comfortably do this, then place pillows under your chest, which will decrease strain to the shoulders and neck. Squeeze your shoulder blades together, then raise your elbows slightly (about 1/4 to 1/2 inch—higher is not better). Focus on using your scapular muscles, rather than your shoulder muscles, to raise your elbows. When doing this correctly, you will feel tension between the scapula and the spine rather than in the shoulder joint. Hold for 3–5 breaths, then lower your elbows while maintaining the scapulae contraction. Finally, relax the scapulae back down. Perform 5–10 repetitions.

COMMON ERRORS

- If you experience pain in your shoulder, be sure your elbows are not rising higher than your wrists. Put more pillows under your chest, so you begin with your arms in a more relaxed position.
- If your head arches back, relax your neck and allow your scapula muscles to work. Be sure to maintain a lengthened neck.

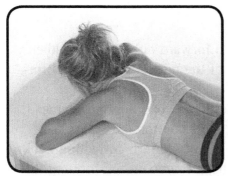
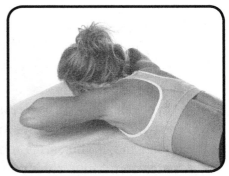

Trapezius Strengthening, start position   Trapezius Strengthening, end position

ARM SLIDES

This exercise restores normal biomechanics and strengthens key muscles involved in rotating, elevating, and stabilizing your shoulder blades. I usually begin this as a single-arm exercise to help focus on one arm at a time. I've broken it down into a movement phase and a strengthening phase. Begin strengthening only after you have mastered the movement.

THE FIXING YOU METHOD—MOVEMENT

Stand a few inches from the wall, so you can comfortably place your elbows and the pinky sides of your hands on the wall as shown below. Be sure your neck is not extended but is instead lengthened at the base of the skull.

Slide your hand up the wall into a diagonal direction away from you (if you are doing this with two arms, then they will create a V-shape). When your elbow is level with your shoulders, shrug your shoulders up to assist in elevating your scapulae. If you have difficulty knowing whether the upper trapezius muscle is working, tap it with your other hand to see whether it is firm from contracting and to help develop your awareness of this muscle. Continue shrugging your shoulders as your arms slide up. Remember, a large part of fixing the shoulder blade is that it must rotate approximately 60 degrees and abduct while the arm is raising (see Landmark 3: Scapular Rotation at 60 Degrees, p. 48). Visualize your scapula rotating under your arm as it rises—in effect supporting the arm in the overhead position. Stop before you feel any pain, and hold for 5 breaths. Slide your arm down while continuing to shrug your shoulder up toward your ear. This activates and strengthens a lengthened or weak upper trapezius muscle. Once your elbow has slid down to about shoulder height again, you can begin to relax the shoulder blade by slowly releasing the shrug. Perform 5–10 repetitions. Your arm should be pain free and able to fully slide up the wall with elevated scapula.

Common Errors

- Pain in your shoulder may be caused by several errors. Your elbows may be rotating out too much (**internal rotation**), causing shoulder pain (see *Fixing You: Shoulder & Elbow Pain*). You may not be resting your arm on the wall enough. Check to see that your shoulders are elevating at the right time—when your elbows are level with your shoulders—and that they continue to shrug up while the arm stretches upward. Stop at or prior to pain.

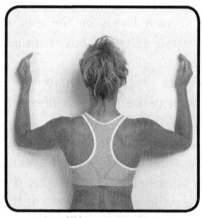

Arm Slides, start position

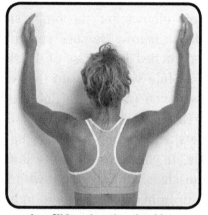

Arm Slides, elevating shoulders

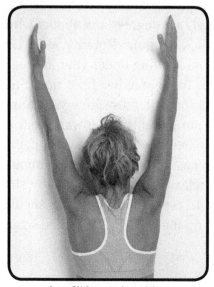

Arm Slides, end position

THE FIXING YOU METHOD—STRENGTHENING

Once your arms are fully elevated, squeeze your scapulae together to lift your hands off the wall by only 1/4 to 1/2 inch—more is not better. Be sure to use your scapulae to lift your hands off as opposed to your shoulder muscles. Lifting with the shoulder muscles may cause pain in the shoulders, whereas squeezing the scapulae together should not.

COMMON ERRORS

- Pain in your shoulders may be caused by using your shoulder muscles instead of your scapulae to lift your hands off the wall. Perform as a single-arm exercise first, and reach behind you with the other hand to feel your scapular muscles engage and lift your arm off the wall.
- Neck pain may result if you extend your head to assist in lifting the arm off the wall. Do not allow this to happen.

HAND ON HEAD

This exercise activates the upper trapezius muscle to elevate your shoulder blade and relax the levator scapula. I've found this to be a useful exercise for nagging neck and shoulder pain, and it can be done almost anywhere.

THE FIXING YOU METHOD

Simply place your hand on top of your head. Relax your arm. Feel that your shoulder is slightly elevated when in this position, and that the upper trapezius muscle is activated to hold up your shoulder. You can be sure the trapezius is activated by feeling it with your other hand, making sure it is firm from contracting. Be sure your head is in good alignment—do not let it side-bend or rotate to either side. Let the weight of your arm rest on your head. Neck pain should be relieved almost instantly if it is originating from the shoulder blade. Only one repetition is necessary to relieve pain. Hold for 30–60 seconds, then relax. When you lower your arm back down, keep the upper trapezius contracted until your arm is all the way down to your side; this helps strengthen and train the upper trapezius muscle. You may feel that your shoulder is resting slightly higher than it was before performing the exercise.

COMMON ERRORS

- Pain in your shoulder might be caused by some **impingement** at the shoulder joint due to improper scapular mechanics. In this case, try bringing your elbow forward so it is pointing in front of you. If this still hurts, then perhaps you are not adequately contracting the upper trapezius muscle. Tap it to connect your awareness to the muscle.

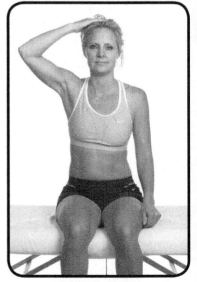

Hand On Head

SIDE-LYING ARM SLIDES

This exercise restores normal range of motion to your shoulder and strengthens key scapular and rotator cuff muscles responsible for **external rotation** of the arm. Again, I've broken this down into a movement part and a strengthening part. Please begin strengthening only after you have mastered the movement. The elbow only needs to slide up a couple inches above the shoulder joint.

THE FIXING YOU METHOD—MOVEMENT

Lie on your side, resting your top arm on pillows so that your arm is roughly at the same height as your shoulder joint. Be sure the scapula is sitting 3 inches from your spine when beginning and upon returning to the start position. If you are still having trouble knowing where your shoulder blade is sitting, then have a friend or therapist check your shoulder for you. With your thumb pointed to the ceiling, slide your hand and elbow along the pillow until your elbow is positioned 2 or 3 inches above your shoulder joint. Be sure your elbow stays on the pillows and your wrist doesn't lower to the floor while sliding your arm. Instead, your wrist should be level with your elbow. When your elbow reaches shoulder level, shrug your shoulder toward your ear to activate the trapezius muscle. Hold the position for 5 breaths and return to the start position. Perform 5–10 repetitions.

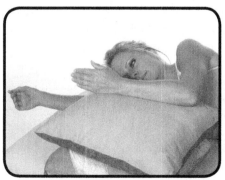
Side-lying Arm Slides, start position

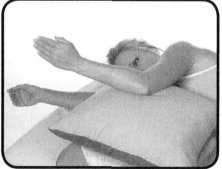
Side-lying Arm Slides, end position

Common Errors

- Pain in your shoulder might be caused by your wrist dropping down toward the floor or your elbow lifting off the pillows. Also, the scapula may not be in its ideal position 3 inches from the spine. Check your form to avoid these errors. Keep your arm heavy on the pillow as you slide the arm up into a pain-free overhead position. Slide your arm within a pain-free range of motion. Do not push through pain to achieve the desired range of motion.

The Fixing You Method—strengthening

Once in the overhead position, squeeze your scapula to your spine to raise your arm from the pillow. Your arm does not need to lift completely off the pillow; you only need to remove its weight from the pillow. Keep your wrist level with your elbow at all times. Hold for 5 breaths. Relax your arm back into the pillow by allowing the scapula to lower it. Slide your arm back down to the start position and perform 5–10 repetitions.

Common Errors

- Pain in your shoulder might be caused by excessive rotation of the arm bone due to your wrist dropping down toward the floor or your elbow rising off the floor. Pain may also result if the shoulder blade is not stabilizing but is instead moving excessively while lifting your arm. Be sure your elbow does not rise off the pillow higher than your wrist. Make sure you use your scapular muscles to raise your arm rather than your shoulder muscles.

ARM WAVES

This exercise helps restore normal range of motion to your shoulder joint and is therefore a powerful tool for fixing shoulder and neck pain issues. By restoring normal range of motion, arm movements will work independently of the scapulae and, therefore, diminish neck involvement when the arm is moving. Internal range of motion should be approximately 70 degrees (fingers touching the floor with wrist bent) and external range of motion should be approximately 90 degrees (arm resting on the floor).

THE FIXING YOU METHOD—INTERNAL ROTATION

Lie on your back with your knees supported or bent. Be sure your lower back is comfortable. Rest your arm on the floor, as shown, so your arm is at a 90-degree angle to your trunk. If your shoulder pops up off the floor, then prop your elbow up on a towel or pillow to allow the shoulder to sink down to the floor more easily.

Place your opposite hand on the shoulder you're exercising to monitor the shoulder joint. It should not pop up during the exercise. Slowly allow your hand to rotate forward and downward toward the table. Keep the shoulder down, and stop if it rises up into your monitoring hand. Allow your hand to rest in the down position for about 30 to 60 seconds, feeling the stretch in the top or back of your shoulder. It may be helpful to allow your arm to rest on a pillow in this position in order to completely relax your shoulder and allow it to stretch. Return to the start position, keeping your shoulder down. Repeat while visualizing the muscles in the back of your shoulder lengthening to allow your hand to drift down to the table. Do not push your hand down—this will make your shoulder pop up. This must be a passive exercise. Hold for 30 to 60 seconds and perform 2–5 repetitions. If you do not experience any pain, you can attach a 1- to 3-pound weight to your wrist to help stretch your arm.

> If your hand is at the side of your body facing your thigh, then **internally rotating** your arm will result in your palm facing behind your body.

Common Errors

- If your shoulder pops up immediately when moving your arm, increase the thickness of the padding under your elbow until you can comfortably perform the exercise and feel a stretch. Or decrease the angle of your shoulder to your trunk from 90 degrees to 70 or 60 degrees—whatever allows your shoulder to stay down. As you improve, work toward sliding your arm to a 90-degree position. You could also try the modified version of this stretch while lying on your side (see below).
- Pain in your shoulder when moving your arm may indicate that you are trying too hard to push your hand down. Relax and let gravity help you instead. Find a point where you can feel a stretch without pain.

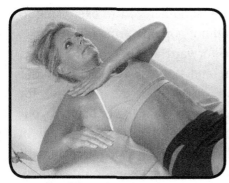 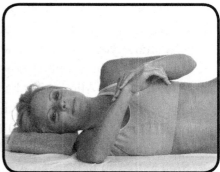

Arm Waves, internal rotation   Arm Waves, modified to side-lying

The Fixing You Method—internal rotation modified to side-lying

This is a good alternative for those with very tight shoulders. Lie on your right side with your right arm on the floor at a 90-degree angle from your body. Bend your elbow 90 degrees, so your hand is pointed up toward the ceiling. With your left hand, slowly and gently help your right hand rotate forward, down toward the floor. Stop once you feel the stretch in the back of your shoulder. Hold for 30–60 seconds and perform 2–5 repetitions.

THE FIXING YOU METHOD—EXTERNAL ROTATION

This is usually easier for most people. While lying on your back with your arm at a 90-degree angle to your trunk as in the **internal rotation** variation, allow your raised hand to rotate backward instead of forward. Your shoulder typically will not rise up in this direction, so you will not need to monitor it. Stop if you experience pain. If this is painful, place a pillow under your hand at the point where you can feel a stretch without pain in order to relax the shoulder muscles. As your muscles stretch out, you can remove the pillow and/or slide your arm upward as shown in the picture below. Hold for 30 to 60 seconds and perform 2–5 repetitions.

> If your palm is at the side of your body facing your thigh, then **externally rotating** your arm will result in your palm facing forward.

COMMON ERRORS

- If you experience pain in your shoulder, place thicker pillows under your elbow until you can feel a stretch with no shoulder pain. Slide your elbow down from the 90-degree position to your side, and attempt the movement again. After your shoulder loosens up, gradually move back into 90 degrees of abduction.

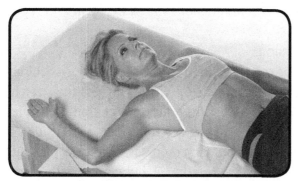

Arm Waves, external rotation

LATISSIMUS DORSI STRETCH

This exercise restores the latissimus dorsi to its normal length. This muscle originates in the lower back and inserts into the upper arm. When tight, it can alter the mechanics of the back, arm, and shoulder and therefore the neck. Normal shoulder range of motion is 170 to 180 degrees of **flexion**. Your arm should almost be able to rest on the table above your head.

THE FIXING YOU METHOD

Lie on your back with your knees bent so that your lower back remains flat; this anchors one end of the latissimus dorsi muscle so you can achieve a better stretch. Use your abdominal muscles to maintain a flat back as you raise your arms overhead, leading with your thumbs as in the picture. Be sure the back of your neck remains lengthened and does not move into **extension**. Feel the stretch in your armpit, ribs, lower back, or upper arm. Make sure your lower back stays down.

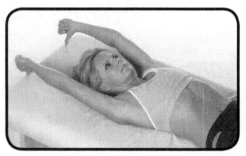

Latissimus Dorsi Stretch

If you have back extension problems, you may experience back pain if your back is allowed to arch up (see *Fixing You: Back Pain*). Hold for 5 breaths or longer. Perform 2–5 repetitions.

COMMON ERRORS

- If you experience pain in the top of your shoulder, begin the exercise again, and stop when you feel the stretch but before you feel pain. Support your arm on a pillow while stretching. Position your arm slightly further out to the side.
- Pain in the shoulder could also indicate that the arm bone needs to rotate. Rotating it outward usually decreases pain. You can gradually rotate it back in as you progress the stretch.

CHEST STRETCH

This exercise stretches the chest muscles that attach to the inner part of the upper arm. When these muscles become tight, they can affect how the shoulder blade rests and moves. You should be able to rest your arm 90 to 120 degrees from your trunk with your palms up, as shown below.

THE FIXING YOU METHOD

Lie on your back with your knees bent to flatten your lower back. Bring your arms out to the side at 90 degrees from your trunk, as shown. Hold for 5 breaths or longer. Be sure your lower back remains flat and does not arch. Relax, then repeat. Slide your arms up to 120 degrees, and stretch there as well. Perform 2–5 repetitions.

COMMON ERRORS

- If you experience pain in your shoulder, place pillows or towels under your arm or wrist to decrease the strain on your shoulder.

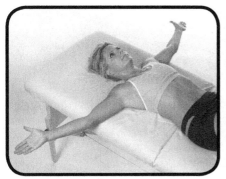
Chest Stretch, start position

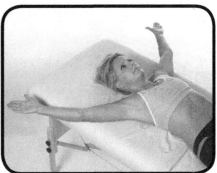
Chest Stretch, end position

CONCLUSION

Neck pain and headaches can be difficult to correct for patients and health care practitioners alike due to the complexity of the structures involved. The scrutiny of damaged structures such as vertebral disks, ligaments, vertebrae, or nerves has traditionally been the focus of neck pain treatment with surgery, traction, ultrasound, manipulation, or other interventions used to target these obviously damaged areas. *Fixing You: Neck Pain & Headaches* introduces a major component of neck function and treatment that is often overlooked: the Fixing You approach addresses overall neck *function* rather than treating damaged structures. This is based on my observation that these structures are often damaged because of poor function, rather than function being impaired due to damaged structures. A thorough examination of the shoulder blade is key to assessing and correcting overall neck function with the Fixing You approach. Shoulder blade function, by virtue of its direct muscular attachments to the neck, is a primary contributor to neck pain and headaches. Correcting your shoulder blade's resting and movement dynamics can be a key component of fixing stubborn neck pain, including pain caused by accidents or injuries. My experience has shown that correcting function eliminates neck pain and headaches in most patients—even in the presence of structural problems, such as degenerated disks or bulging disks.

A recurring theme I hear from new clients is that they do not believe they can lead fully pain-free lives because of an injury or a structural diagnosis. It's no wonder after seeing MRIs or X-rays of their condition that show a clear structural problem that "must be" causing the pain and speaking to specialists who reinforce the idea that a structural problem equals a permanent issue. After reading my clients' stories in this book, however, you've discovered that even with these conditions, you can be pain free. This is because the pain isn't necessarily caused by those damaged structures; instead, it is often a result of poor function that has led to structural damage. This is also true of other chronic aches and pains elsewhere in the body. My Fixing You book series can be ordered through the website and covers many common chronic and recurring injuries, aches, and pains. The Fixing You approach is designed to improve your body's biomechanics by correcting movement dysfunctions, retraining your body to restore it to its optimal state— healthy and pain free.

Remember, you can also watch video clips of the assessments and exercises on our website, **www.FixingYou.net**. I strongly encourage you to take advantage of these visual tools to ensure that you are performing the exercises correctly and to further empower yourself by learning more about how to take the best care of your body. I would also like to extend an invitation for you to share your experiences with me, whether good or bad. My intention is to help as many people as possible. Your suggestions will help me improve future editions. Please feel free to share your success stories or questions. You can reach me at **Rick@FixingYou.net**.

I encourage you to believe in your ability to take control of your body and commit to the process of fixing yourself. You will learn a great deal about your habits and your strengths and weaknesses—and that you can get past limitations once you begin. Stay positive, and keep paying attention to your body. Own the power to fix yourself—you have it within you!

GLOSSARY

abducting
Moving out to the side, away from the midline of the body. For instance, when moving your arm out to the side, your arm is abducting.

abduction
A position that results from abducting an appendage. For example, an arm held out to the side is said to be in abduction.

anterior
In front or forward; opposite of posterior. For instance, the nose is anterior to the ears.

cervical spine
The neck portion of the spine composed of the cervical vertebrae.

cervical vertebrae—See vertebrae

clavicle
Collarbone that attaches from the trunk at the sternum to the shoulder at the acromion (see **scapula**).

degenerated disk (degenerative disk disease)
A condition in which the disks between vertebrae loose their integrity and shock-absorbing properties, and the disk becomes thinner.

disk (intervertebral disk)
A cushion between vertebrae that provides spacing and shock-absorbing properties. Stresses placed on a disk can change its shape, forming bulges or tears.

disk bulge
A structural diagnosis wherein the disk between two vertebrae has become misshapen, forming a bulge at one area.

disk herniation
A structural diagnosis wherein the disk tissue tears and a portion of the inner disk material escapes the disk's confines.

depressed scapula
A scapula that rests lower than it should on the trunk. This typically also involves problems with elevation, rotation, and abduction of the scapula.

extending
The act of straightening a joint or reversing a flexed position.

extension
Describes a position that is extended relative to neutral or flexion.

external rotation
Rotating the anterior surface of a bone or joint away from the midline of the body; also referred to as lateral rotation.

flexing
The act of bending a joint; the opposite of extending.

flexion
Describes a position that is flexed relative to neutral or extension.

functional problem
When the body does not move correctly due to weakness, impaired range of motion, previous injury, or habitual movement patterns. Functional problems typically create pain and may cause physical changes to tissues.

herniated disk—See disk herniation.

humerus
The upper arm bone. The head of the humerus (humeral head) fits into the shoulder socket to form the shoulder joint.

hypermobile joint
A joint that has too much motion, which may or may not be well controlled, is hypermobile. A hypermobile joint often occurs near a hypomobile joint.

hypomobile joint
A joint that has too little motion. When a joint does not move well, other joints above or below it typically must compensate by becoming hypermobile in order to achieve functional movement.

impingement
Pinched or compressed tissue, usually between two bones. For instance, a nerve may become impinged if it is pinched between two vertebrae.

inferior angle—See scapula.

internal rotation
Rotating the anterior surface of a bone or joint toward the midline of the body; also referred to as medial rotation.

levator scapula
A muscle that originates at the shoulder blade and inserts into the first four cervical vertebrae; it can contribute to excessive movements of the cervical spine.

medial rotation—See internal rotation.

movement dysfunction
A way of moving that is unnatural to optimal biomechanics and causes pain; also referred to as movement fault.

Pilates
A method of exercising using springs for tension; it can also be taught as a mat class, similar to yoga. Pilates can be a safe method for strengthening the body in the presence of an injury.

posterior
Behind or in back of; the opposite of anterior. For instance, the heel of the foot is posterior to the toes.

scapula
Also known as the shoulder blade. This triangular bone articulates with the arm bone to form the shoulder joint. Scapular function is important to preventing or fixing shoulder and neck injuries.

> **vertebral border:** The border that is closest to and runs roughly parallel to the spine.

> **coracoid process:** A bony prominence to which the pectoralis minor muscle and the short head of the biceps muscle attaches.

> **acromion:** Forms the "roof" of the shoulder joint and articulates with the clavicle.

> **inferior angle:** The bottom corner of the scapula.

> **spine:** A ridge along the scapula that terminates in the acromion. The infraspinatus, teres major, and teres minor muscles originate below the spine; the supraspinatus muscle originates above the spine. The spine is palpated to assess scapular position on the trunk.

structural diagnosis
A diagnosis describing a physical change in the body such as a bulging disk or arthritis.

thoracic vertebra—See vertebrae.

trapezius
A large muscle group of the shoulder, neck, and upper back. The trapezius muscle is important to shoulder (and therefore neck) function and is divided into three zones:

upper: Originates at the base of the skull and down a thick ligament connecting to the spine. It inserts into the clavicle and acromion of the scapula. This portion elevates the scapula during arm movements, stabilizes the scapula during adduction, and assists with rotation.

mid: Originates from thoracic vertebrae 1 to 5 and inserts into the acromion and spine of the scapula. This portion adducts and stabilizes during scapular rotation.

lower: Originates from thoracic vertebrae 6 to 12 and inserts into the spine of the scapula. This portion depresses and rotates the scapula.

trigger point
A hypersensitive point or nodule in muscle that, when pressed, elicits pain in a distant site.

vertebrae (singular: vertebra)
The bones that comprise the spine. They are divided into three sections.

cervical: The neck region. There are seven cervical vertebrae.

thoracic: The upper trunk region where ribs attach. There are twelve thoracic vertebrae.

lumbar: The lower spine region composed of five vertebrae.

vertebral border—See scapula.

REFERENCES

Introduction opening quote:
Nechis, Barbara. 1993. *Watercolor from the Heart.* New York: Watson-Guptill Publications.

Section 1 opening quote:
Yogananda, Paramahansa. 1997. *Journey to Self-Realization.* Los Angeles, CA: Self-Realization Fellowship.

Section 2 opening quote:
Chopra, Deepak. 1993. *Creating Affluence: Wealth Concsciousness in the Field of All Possibilities.* San Rafael, CA: New World Library.

Section 3 opening quote:
Campbell, Joseph. 1991. *The Joseph Campbell Companion: Reflections on the Art of Living.* Ed. Diane K. Osbon. New York: HarperCollins.

Kendall, Florence, Elizabeth McCreary, and Patricia Provance. 1993. *Muscles Testing and Function.* Fourth edition. Baltimore, MD: Williams & Wilkins.

Sahrmann, Shirley A. 2002. *Diagnosis and Treatment of Movement Impairment Syndromes.* St. Louis, MO: Mosby.

ABOUT THE AUTHOR

Rick Olderman MSPT, CPT

Following graduation in 1996 from the nationally ranked Krannert School of Physical Therapy at the University of Indianapolis, I practiced at a small sports and orthopedic clinic in Cortez, Colorado. Because the clinic had a small gym attached, I was able to progress patients to a higher functional level than if I were in a typical clinic. This unique model influenced me to consider personal training. I discovered that setting up therapeutic training programs for my patients helped them as much or more than any intervention I would perform manually.

I moved to Denver in 1999 and began working as a physical therapist and personal trainer at an exclusive health club, The Athletic Club at Denver Place. While there, I continued to experiment with blending rehabilitation and personal training and added Pilates to my skill set. Within just a few months, I became the top-producing employee at the club. I held that position for the next four years until I opened my own studio/clinic.

In addition to providing individual client services, I also lead corporate seminars for injury prevention and correction. My focus on teaching employees the fundamentals of injury mechanics and practical ways to correct them has made me an effective force in changing corporate thinking about injuries, injury prevention, ergonomics, and fitness programs. I believe education is the key. I find that if you teach someone how the body works and why they experience pain, most people will be more diligent in helping themselves. No one wants to be in pain.

I am an active member of the American Physical Therapy Association, and I continue to explore combined rehabilitation and fitness techniques through professional development and continuing education. I live and work in Denver, Colorado with my wife and two young children.

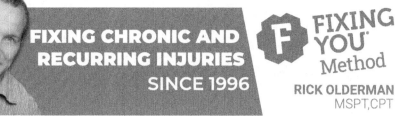
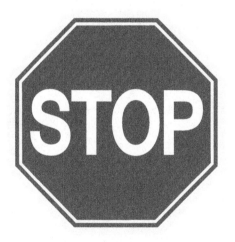

Made in the USA
Middletown, DE
10 December 2022

17944415R00056